Don't Touch Your Toes!

The right way to total fitness

By **Roger E. Greeley**
with **Constantine Nicholas, M.D.**
Member, American Academy of Orthopedic Surgeons

Visuals by **Dr. David Curl,** Oak Woods Media

Rand McNally & Company
Chicago • New York • San Francisco

All photographs were taken by Dr. David Curl except for those on pages 74–81, which were by Elliott H. McCleary

Printed in the United States of America
by Rand McNally & Company

First printing, 1982

Library of Congress Catalog Card Number: 82-60184

To KPG, my greatest companion

Contents

How to Use This Fitness Manual

First of all, read it, please!

This is not simply an exercise book. It is a fitness book with a different point of view, a view that challenges outdated ideas of fitness. So please first read the book in its entirety, including the exercises. Then go to the illustrated "Daily Exercises for Fitness" chapter and begin.

All the exercises are suitable for the beginner except the few marked intermediate and advanced. Perform every one of them in the order given.

Above all, be faithful to all aspects of the program outlined here, including the tips for proper body maintenance. Your physical well-being depends on your mental commitment to achieve fitness. Maintain a firm psychological commitment and a relaxed attitude that embraces patience with yourself.

FITness Not FEATness!

"I weigh too much."
"I shouldn't smoke."
"I have been drinking more than I used to."
"I don't sleep as soundly as I'd like."
"Why am I so tense?"
"Are these headaches caused by tension?"
"My nerves are shot."
"I take tranquilizers too often now."

These are concerns of millions of Americans who are struggling at home, at work, and at play to live happier lives.

Basic requirements for happiness include achievement of a proper perspective of one's life and a good balance between work and play.

Few people suggest that one's physical well-being does not contribute to one's state of mind. Often we are down because of a rotten cold, the flu, or a headache.

At the same time, as psychologists have pointed out, physical well-being is very definitely influenced by one's state of mind and emotions. In this regard, so-called "sexercises" are, at best, suspect. If ever the mental state took precedence over the physical, it is in this matter of sexual performance. Let one's heart and head be in tune, and general fitness will be enough.

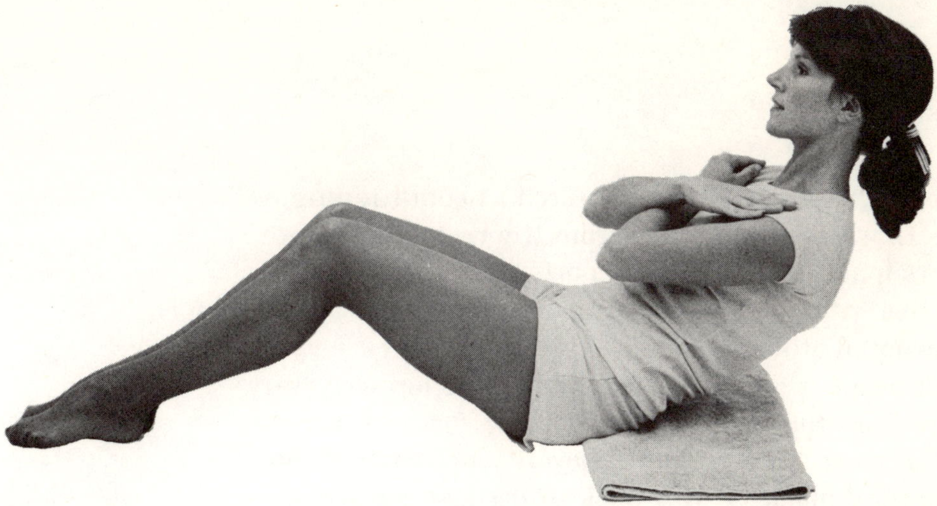

As a result of this interdependence between the two states of being, there has been an enormous proliferation of programs, products, and activities to promote inner peace, happiness, and feeling fit. To list but a few that have gained prominence in recent years reveals the American obsession with feeling good: yoga, biofeedback, TM (transcendental meditation), TA (transactional analysis), hundreds of health spas, jogging, the Royal Canadian Air Force exercise manual, the Stillman and Atkins diets, Weight Watchers, home exercisers, gyms, twist-boards, springs, elastics, weights, wheels, machines of all sizes and promises, biorhythms, astrology, yogurt, vitamin E, and countless others that would seem to preclude the publication of yet another book on personal fitness. Not so.

The fundamental premise of this book represents a radical departure from the predominant emphasis of traditional physical education. Here you will find exercises designed to prepare you for and protect you from the stresses, strains, and demands of normal living. They give you "functional fitness."

Functional fitness is not, for example, an athlete's watered-down conditioning program. It does not involve a series of routines in which the ultimate goal is the mastery of certain skills and graded feats.

For decades the tail has wagged the dog in physical

education. This has generally resulted in conditioning routines that have been taken from the regimens of those who participate in competitive sports. There are more nonathletes in this nation than there are genuine amateur or professional athletes.

Most people want to feel good and function well every day more than they want to be stellar performers in a particular sport. That is simply beyond the reach of the overwhelming majority. Way back in the last century a nonathlete (attorney-lecturer Robert Ingersoll) made a very astute observation concerning physical education. He wrote: "The gymnast or athlete should seek for health as the student should seek for truth. When athletics degenerate into mere personal contests, they become dangerous, because the contestants lose sight of health." Today, many people are partially crippled or restricted in their daily activities by severe injuries incurred in the kind of competitive sports that often place the individual's health second to the team's success.

A basic assumption of this book is that FITness, not FEATness, should be the first concern of all men and women. Therefore, this program appeals first to the nonathlete, the mature adult who wants to lose weight, stop smoking, wants more pep and stamina, but is not happy with traditional competitive calisthenics. He or she may not have the time or the inclination to get involved in a class, group, or club, but may well prefer the privacy and economy of exercising at home. Your personal schedule may not provide for regularly scheduled visits to a spa, gym, or exercise class. This program can be done in the home and elsewhere throughout each day.

A second assumption of this program is that each and every exercise should relate as closely as possible to the performance of common manual tasks. Each of us finds it necessary to lift, sit, walk, iron, wash, sweep, rake, shovel, mop, shower, bathe, hoe, weed, mow, launder, shop, rearrange furniture, build a fire in the fireplace, set up card tables, and do countless other jobs that call for strength and flexibility. Few men appreciate the heavy physical demands of keeping house until the woman of the house is felled by the flu! The manner in which many simple household and office tasks are done determines how you will feel at the end of the day. Many of the jobs that we do each day are done incorrectly; that is, we expend more energy and incur greater strain than we need to until we learn the proper how-to's!

Unfortunately, much of what has passed for sound exercise and good conditioning has not been that at all. In fact, some of the most traditional exercises are downright destructive. The title of this book is no accident; it is a prescription. It means exactly what it says. Touching your toes without bending the knees is still regarded as a measure of fitness by millions of people who have been raised with this belief. Consider for a moment whether toe touching relates to any activity that you will encounter any day of your life. It does not! Therefore, it must be concluded that toe touching is an end in itself; it is a FEAT. Unless you are anxious to get into the *Guinness Book of World Records* for some aspect of toe touching, it has no value beyond being a FEAT. FEATness is not FITness. Many an orthopedic surgeon recommends dropping toe touching and related exercises altogether. Does this mean that orthopedists are not interested in fitness and flexibility? Of course not. It is precisely because of their interest that they criticize strongly those routines that are potentially injurious to man, woman, and child.

My resource person, the coauthor of this program, is an orthopedic surgeon, Dr. Constantine Nicholas, who was the first person to call to my attention the fallacies of traditional conditioning which I, as a former physical education instructor, was guilty of teaching and doing myself. After an accident while vacuuming the house one day, I was forced to reexamine my whole approach to fitness. In consultation with Dr. Nicholas, I worked out the program in this manual.

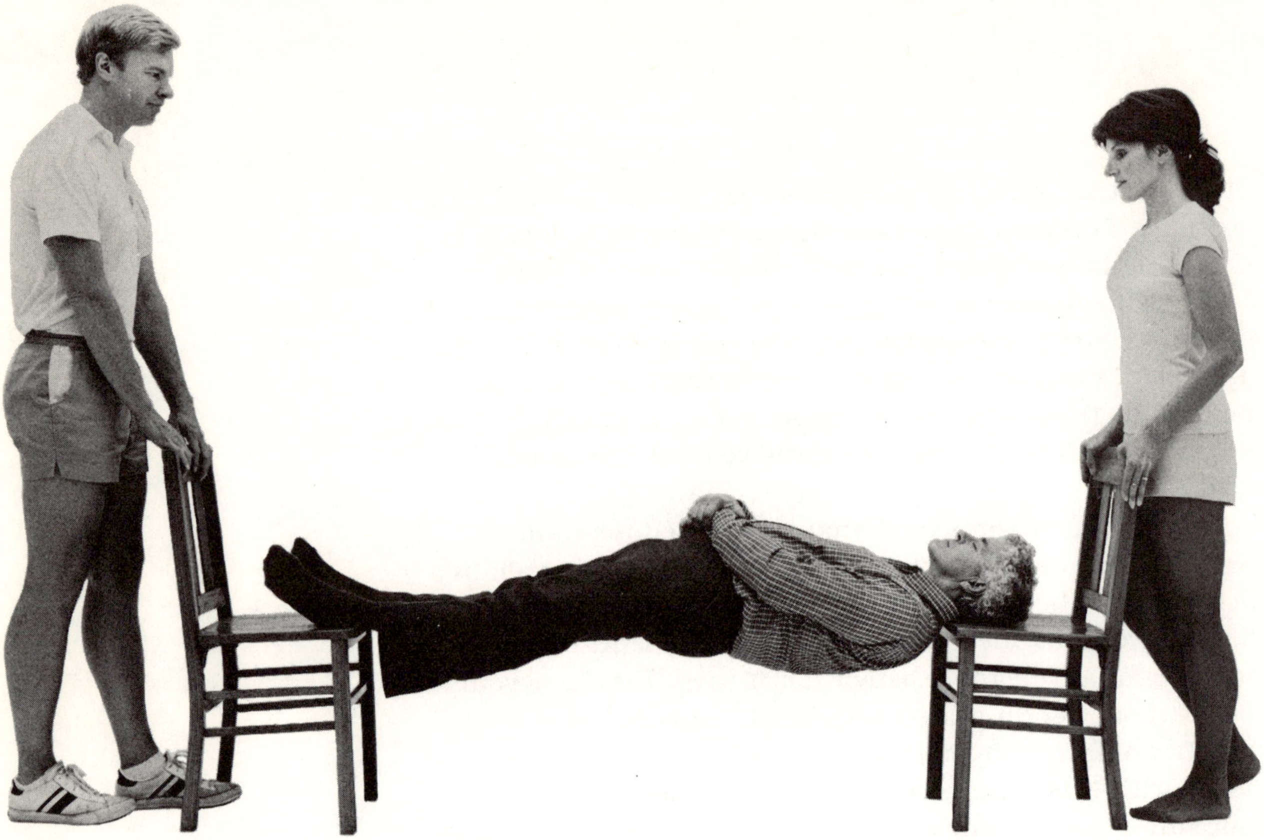

The author (between chairs) demonstrates what this book is *not* about: FEATness. Whether or not you can perform certain athletic feats is no more relevant to your daily life than the ability to do this silly stunt. The exercises in this book make you fit for the common tasks of daily life.

Some of today's more progressive instructors in PE have dropped most of the detrimental routines from conditioning programs. The fact that they are still being performed in many schools, spas, and gyms means that the word must get around if we are going to protect the young and improve our approach to fitness. Here is the key consideration: Will we put FITness ahead of FEATness? That is, are we to be more concerned with the ability to function well throughout life than we are in mastering certain sports-related skills, feats, tests, and contests?

The two need not be mutually exclusive. What is clear, however, is that participation in sports does not accompany most people all the days of their lives. After age 30, participation in weekend games and sports activities is *not* the pathway to fitness. What is more likely is that those who are fit will be able to enjoy their organized sports activities after passing their 30th birthday. For the mature person, sports activities can provide relaxation and recreation, but realistically, these activities cannot ensure overall fitness.

Fitness is a condition resulting from one's daily awareness and actions. Fitness is a companion that walks with us from cradle to grave. It is entirely possible that a person can be exceptionally fit and yet not be distinguished in performance of specific sports or feats. Conversely, there are some who can perform well in sports but who truly are not functionally fit. They may be overweight, dependent upon drugs, tobacco or alcohol, worried, insomniac, or tense.

We believe that if one must choose between FEATness and FITness, there is, in reality, no choice. We all want to be fit, to enjoy life, to perform throughout each day in a comfortable and effective manner. We want to look well and feel good! Unfortunately, surrounded as we are in a society that idolizes youth, we tend to demand the impossible: eternal youth. We confuse fitness with being young again.

As he was approaching his 60s, Robert Ingersoll was asked, "How is it that you have been able to age so gracefully?" He replied, "It is very hard to live a great while without getting old, and it is hardly worthwhile to die early just to keep young." Functional fitness accepts the realism of the aging process; it does not lie down and give up but urges the individual to maximize his or her fitness within the limits imposed by nature.

Surely, the results are not often good when, after 20 years of idleness, the 45-year-old takes up jogging and overdoes it. At the same time, those at 35, 40, or older who feel they are past their need and ability to exercise are equally unthinking and unaware of their true potential.

We know that this program offers every mature adult a pathway to functional fitness. To be alive remains the highest miracle of the natural universe. Enhance that living by sensible eating, adequate rest, and exercise for fitness, fitness to function every day of your life. Enjoy!

Don't Touch Your Toes!

(And Other Warnings)

Of all the warm-up exercises performed in the typical gym class, toe touching is surely the one that stands first in the litany of useless feats. There is no sound physical reason for trying to touch your toes without bending your knees. On the other hand, there are several very good reasons why you should *not* try to touch your toes without bending your knees.

If your gym teacher or coach was really high on toe touching, he might well have singled out for a demonstration the class contortionist who could literally put his or her elbows on the floor. After a suitable pause for the "oohs" and "ahhs" to subside, the coach might then comment on what *real* dedication and hard work can produce. It is a tribute to the natural conformity and fear in students that only rarely did a student ever inquire as to why the coach couldn't perform this feat!

The response to the elbow-to-floor demonstration is predictable. A few students might emulate this paragon; the majority, however, simply shake their heads in bewildered dismay, muttering something about "freaks."

Without a doubt, we are impressed with such a demonstration, for it is a unique and unusual feat to touch one's elbows to the floor while keeping the legs straight. It is entirely fair, however, for a student to ask, "What good is

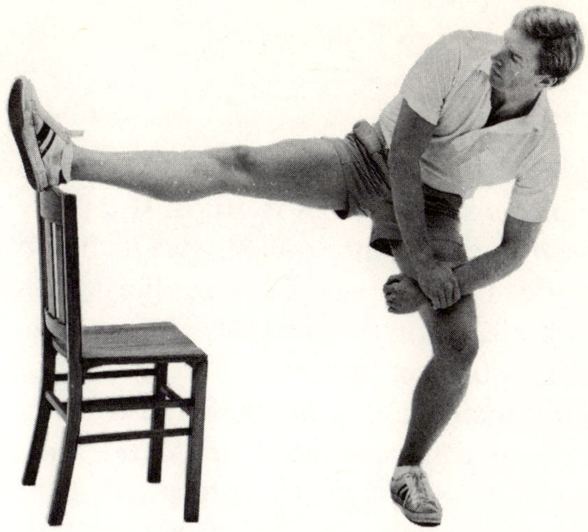

that, Coach? How is it going to help me?" Now, if the coach is truly honest he will not have a valid answer. It has certain appeal to those who like that kind of a feat. But it does the body no good and for many of us is downright injurious.

Basically, what is wrong with toe touching is that it puts an unnatural and excessive strain on the muscles, ligaments, and nerves of the lower back. In view of the fact that the small of the back and the knees are the two most vulnerable areas for injury, neither should be harmed or exploited for the sake of a FEAT.

Frequently, in defense of toe touching, it is said to be *the* exercise to achieve "suppleness." This, however, really demands a definition as to what constitutes suppleness. The only suppleness of significance is that which relates to function. There are not any logical functions of everyday living that involve one's adopting the posture of a hairpin. The potential danger inherent in toe touching (injury to the lower back) should alone dictate its being discarded.

Another argument for toe touching is that it is good for loosening the hamstrings, the long, large muscles on the backs of the thighs. A simple dancer's exercise for the hamstrings is far more effective and offers no threat to the back at all. This exercise is discussed and pictured in the "Daily Exercises for Fitness" chapter.

Speaking more positively, however, it is what toe touching does *not* do that forces it out of the exercise routine. It does *not* contribute one single useful thing to functional fitness. In fact, it tends to reinforce bad habits in the manner of performing simple tasks. It tends to make us bend our backs instead of our legs.

In summary, toe touching is a worthless yet almost sacrosanct exercise, often viewed as if written in stone. Honestly, you will be better off if you forget it. It is a test of nothing but tradition. You can achieve functional fitness without this feat. In fact, your chances of doing so are greatly enhanced by avoiding toe touching and its related influences on other activities.

The Danger of Sit-Ups

Next, we come to the sit-up. The sit-up is another blue-ribbon feat in the PE Hall of Fame. There are even schools that publicly post the records for number of sit-ups performed (with appropriate sexual discrimination). You may remember yourself, pairing off with a partner who held your feet while you, with hands clasped behind your head, sought to sit up. Repeatedly, you were needled by your partner (often at the coach's urging) to sit up again and again. (Inwardly, you looked forward only to the time when you might hold your partner's feet!)

The coach was always quick to point out that "real athletes don't need anyone to hold their feet down. They've got the kind of intestinal fortitude necessary to do sit-ups *right*!" As far back as President Kennedy's Council on Physical Fitness, the sit-up was condemned for its potential threat to, you guessed it, the lower back.

The claim that the sit-up toughened the abdominal area was, of course, partly true. What went on uncontested was that there might be a better way to toughen the abdominal muscles without subjecting the small of the back to great potential injury.

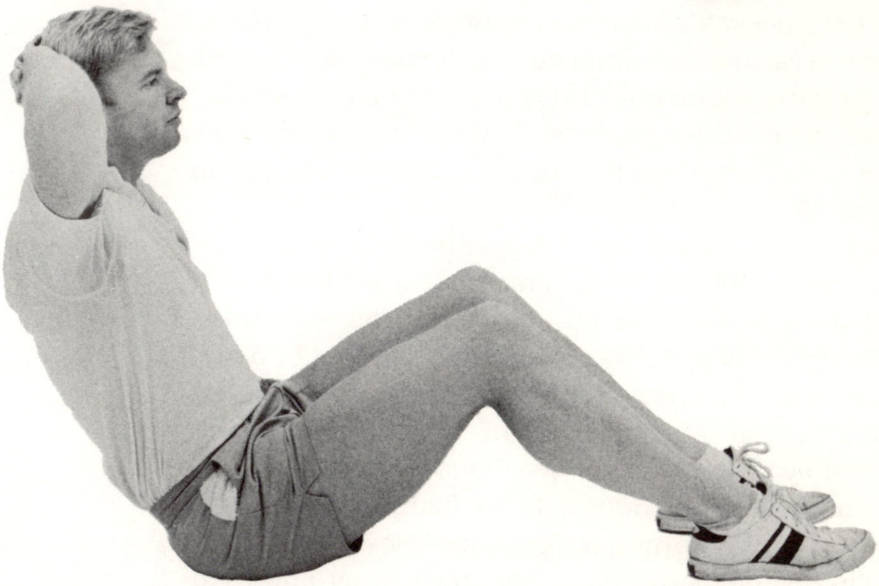

The sitback strengthens abdominal muscles without unduly stressing the lower back.

Basically, the worth of an exercise lies in the specificity it achieves. If you are concerned about the abdominal area, then perform an exercise that will, as far as possible, isolate that particular muscle group. Holding the feet down or hooking them under the bed transfers the stress from the abdominal area to the legs and the back.

The exercise generally recommended today is the "Sitback," which will be described and pictured in the "Daily Exercises for Fitness" chapter. Done correctly, it will do wonders for the abdominal area without any strain to the small of the back.

Exercises that Damage the Knees

Whenever I watch a Johnny Bench or a Carlton Fisk, my knees ache. The baseball catcher's position is a difficult posture for the knees. With the exception of catching, there are not many occasions in which such a "squat" is required in order to perform a function. Do you remember those "All together now, deep knee bends. One—down, two—up," and so on? Rare is the gym class that did not include a period of deep knee bends.

Again, the objections of the orthopedist have finally made a dent on the PE establishment. Deep knee bends have almost disappeared from PE. Where they haven't, they should! Although it is perfectly safe for most people to bend deeply at the knees from time to time during daily activities, there just isn't any argument about the fact that the knees can be injured by repeated deep-knee-bend exercises. This has been well known to orthopedists for many years.

Coaches have often urged the practice known as waddling. That is, one assumes a deep knee squat and then waddles around, demonstrating mobility and, incidentally, no regard for the knees.

So, you can now discard the deep knee bend as well as the traditional sit-up and toe touching. Naturally, the knees and the legs are extremely important in functional fitness, and much attention in this program is devoted to strengthening them. But none of our exercises sacrifice FITness for FEATness.

To Jog or Not?

The great popularity that jogging has enjoyed in recent years would seem to indicate that it is the perfect exercise. This is not necessarily so. Depending on your age, weight, knees, and lower back, jogging could do you more harm than good. Consider the following experiences of a 39-year-old who embarked on a vigorous jogging program because he really didn't want to admit that he would soon be 40.

Ron was dedicated and enthusiastic about jogging. Soon he was jogging a mile, then 2, 3, and even more. He awoke one morning, and when he stepped into the shower he felt sharp pains alongside his shins. Ron had developed what is called "shinsplints." The injury can be painful, prolonged, and quite debilitating. Rest is the best and surest cure. Cortisone has sometimes been used, but this simply masks the symptoms, thus opening the way for additional exacerbation of the tissues.

But Ron, like most Americans, wanted an instant cure. In America, we want "instant" everything: coffee, love, health, fitness, and instant recovery when we are injured or ill. Nearly all muscular injuries, particularly for those over age 30, demand rest and time, or healing will not take place.

Because of his enthusiasm for jogging, Ron tried everything but resting. He ended up on crutches, and a thorough examination revealed a minor disc problem in his lower back, occasioned in part by the pounding that accompanies jogging on a hard surface.

Ron's case is far from unique. Television has brought marathons into our living rooms, and many an armchair athlete sees these as events in which he or she could excel and also lose some weight. There is also the mistaken notion that jogging restores youth. No matter how fast you run, you'll never catch your youth.

Some of us, unfortunately, have an additional worry about jogging, particularly if it is done outdoors in the evening. There is the very distinct danger, in certain populated areas, of criminal assault. This is a grim reality of urban society today.

Why jog? Because it is good exercise for the cardiovascular system—the heart and blood vessels. The heart is a pump made up essentially of muscle, and our arteries are lined with muscle. Every muscle needs exercise. If you want your heart and blood vessels to function well, they must be exercised. If your heart is strong, it will be better able to meet any unusual demands placed upon it, whether caused by strong emotion, running for a bus, or digesting a meal.

There are other ways of performing good cardiovascular exercise without the risks and special demands of jogging. Some alternatives are fast dancing, skipping rope, or that old standby, running in place. My own choice is skipping rope, but you may prefer either of the other two. Whatever exercise you pick, build into it slowly yet vigorously. *Really* dance, skip, or run, and gradually increase the amount of time each day. Of course, if you love jogging and are able to find the time, the place, and the companionship, jogging may be your first choice. If you are a jogger, throw in a little sprint now and then to really tax the cardiovascular system.

Cautions

Anyone who is over age 35, more than 20 pounds overweight, or has a personal or family history of heart trouble should *first consult a physician* before embarking on any vigorous program of cardiovascular exercise.

Do not try to accomplish in a day or a week what you have spent years neglecting! Be patient with yourself, but be faithful to exercise every appropriate opportunity to better your cardiovascular system. Incidentally, running upstairs is much easier for your knees than running downstairs, and it is far more exercise for the heart and lungs.

If you are overweight, the best thing you can do for your heart is to lose the excess weight. Do not seek to "run the fat off." That alone will not work. Proper diet must accompany any attempt to lose weight.

Generally speaking, people who have been overweight and sedentary for some time should not engage in a lot of vigorous exercise until much of the excess weight has been shed. The heart, already taxed by having to maintain all the excess fat, may not be able to handle the sudden additional burden of heavy cardiovascular exercise.

Walking—Effective and Safe

Because walking is such a commonplace, everyday experience, we tend not to think of it as exercise. Wrong! Brisk walking is an outstanding form of exercise. People often ask, "Yeah, but what's your idea of brisk?" Assuming you have normal health, you should strive to walk a mile in 12 to 14 minutes; that's brisk enough. I try to walk at least 3 miles each day for exercise.

The advantage of brisk walking over jogging is that one rarely turns an ankle, tears up a knee, or suffers lower back pains.

Your schedule may not always allow for long walks, but try to compensate for days missed with a simple variation. While walking, particularly when going uphill, recite your favorite poem or prose piece. If you do not know any by heart, here is a good reason to learn one! You will find walking and reciting to be very taxing. Do not become alarmed if at first you seem very breathless after a stanza or two. You will improve with practice.

Your muscles are calling for more oxygen, and you are using much of your air supply for reciting. You are vigorously exercising the whole cardiovascular system when walking and talking. If you are self-conscious about people wondering whether you have joined the "I-talk-to-myself crowd," walk in the woods or in a neighborhood where you are a stranger. If it's cold, you can always put a scarf over your mouth. This also warms the cold air, which is not a bad idea.

Another benefit of walking is that it is a great tension-releasing exercise. Tension headaches tend to disappear after a half hour of brisk walking. You are also away from the telephone and the calls for your attention; it is a time alone to sort things out and to restore the sagging spirit. Yes, it should be enjoyable.

Walk that you may keep the juices flowing.

Walk that you may improve your cardiovascular functions.

Walk that you may reflect and restore.

Walk that you may enjoy achieving FITness.

And lastly,

Walk, there's probably no place to park your car anyway!

Remember, it is in every way, every day, that we make ourselves truly fit and able to function and enjoy life.

Sleep—Good Medicine!

When I was a boy I used to go to my father with my physical complaints. He was an M.D. Invariably, he would say, "Go to bed, you'll be all right in the morning." I recall that his diagnosis was wrong just once. The rest of the time he was right. Part of overall fitness demands proper nutrition along with exercise and sufficient rest—sleep. That sleep should be on a firm or extra-firm mattress or one made firm by a 3/4-inch-thick bedboard, so you sleep on the level and don't wake with a morning backache.

We have long recognized that negative attitudes and feelings affect us negatively. Is it preposterous to suggest that positive attitudes can affect us positively? Try to "psych" yourself up for the things you *can* do that contribute to your personal fitness and feelings of well-being. Do not dwell on the things that are beyond your skills or that discourage you. Instead, truly concentrate on what you *can* do to move toward greater fitness.

With a little effort (and a lot of patience) you can eat properly, celebrate in moderation, stretch and walk regularly, and exercise throughout each day in everything that you do. Take two stairs at a time, walk briskly, breathe deeply, get up and move, stretch, and be active. Most people rust out rather than wear out. We tend to think of exercise as a time apart from our everyday routine. Not so. Exercise is how we eat, celebrate, walk, and do everything throughout each day.

In the next chapter is the most important exercise of all. Chances are you will need it. You've heard of it many times before, and some are depressed when it is presented to them once more. It is a vital aspect of this program and cannot be ignored if you are serious about your fitness. Read this chapter with a love of yourself in mind. Maybe that will make it work to your advantage.

"Basically, what is wrong with toe touching is that it puts an unnatural and excessive strain on the muscles, ligaments, and nerves of the lower back. In view of the fact that the small of the back and the knees are the two most vulnerable areas for injury, neither should be harmed or exploited for the sake of a FEAT."

Body Care

Many people are looking for something *outside* themselves to improve their fitness—a diet pill, for example, or an exercise machine.

You've probably heard the story about the skinny, 98-pound weakling who sent away for the Charles Atlas Dynamic Tension program. After reading the program for six months, the discouraged young man sat down and wrote the following to Mr. Atlas: "I've been on your program for six months. Please send the muscles."

Fitness, like those muscles, is not something outside of you that you purchase or absorb; it is something inside. You must accept responsibility for your own health by utilizing the resources that are in you. They are there, ready to serve you if you will take the time, have the patience, and observe the regimens consistently.

Proper exercise is important for maintaining fitness, but it is only one factor. Other "musts" include diet, nutrition, good posture, and care of the knees and back.

Obesity and Other Hazards

If you are a typical American male or female, the most important exercise for you to do as you begin this program is incredibly simple yet terribly difficult. How can it be both

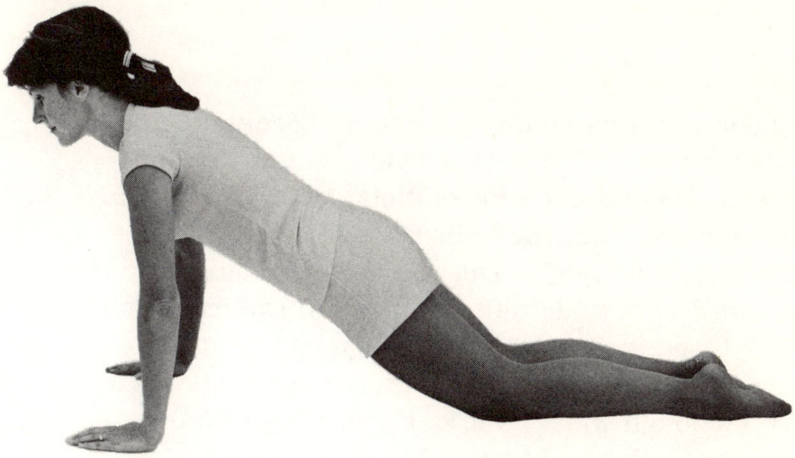

of these at the same time? It is incredibly easy because it involves virtually no expenditure of energy or strength. It is terribly difficult because it demands a total psychological commitment, a great act of will. The exercise: Get up from the dinner table sooner! That's right. At the heart of all sensible exercises is proper weight and nutrition. There is no functional fitness where obesity, modest or great, is a factor.

Nationwide, obesity is one of our greatest health problems. It is the curse of an affluent society. Obesity is largely a psychological problem. It is psychological because no one is forcing another person to eat. The act of overeating is rooted in the individual's attitude about food, eating, and drinking. If you want to achieve total functional fitness, your weight should be 3 to 7 pounds above what it was when you first achieved physical maturity (unless, of course, you were told at age 18 to 21 that you were already overweight).

Unfortunately, many people put on something like a pound every year after they're age 35 (oftentimes before). At such a rate, a person who weighed, let us say 118 pounds when 18 years old will at age 48 weigh 148 pounds and even more. There is no way to achieve functional fitness without maintaining your proper body weight!

This book contains no diets, for it is my contention that the only way to lose and maintain weight is to consume fewer calories. There are dozens of diets. Most physicians will admit, however, that the reduction of calories is the only sure way to lose weight. Did you ever see a survivor of a month-long ordeal in a life raft come aboard the rescue ship looking fat? If you eat less, you will weigh less.

Plan to fall madly in love with water. First of all, few people drink enough water as it is. If you suspect I am endorsing a water diet, forget it. That is not my point. Water is an ideal snack between meals. If you like ice water, use that. Above all, no matter what games you play in regard to your eating, remember you cannot fool your body. Calories do count. If you want to lose weight, cut calories. It is as simple as that. Also, be a little patient with yourself. You didn't put on your weight overnight, and you won't take it off overnight either.

You can achieve your weight-loss goal if you accept the total responsibility for it and do not blame your glands, your upbringing, or the demands of your everyday life. Now and then, doctors determine that a glandular malfunction contributes to obesity, but for every one such case there are many others who claim that glands are the reason for their obesity, when in fact, it's just overeating.

Because we are an affluent society consuming too much of everything, we carry on the same way at the dinner table. It is hard to resist the temptations of overeating. That is why I said that the first exercise is both easy and hard. In the physical sense, it is easy to get up from the table. The psychological discipline, however, is quite another matter.

I am truly sorry not to be able to offer you any instant weight-loss technique as part of this functional fitness program. It is less than honest to pretend to have the instant, magic cure so many people want. Cut calories, period. Some fine diets offer substantial volume yet few calories. Eat slower, eat a lot of virtually no-calorie or low-calorie foods, and you will lose weight.

The philosophy of the organized Weight Watchers program has been very successful for many people. Perhaps you can do what needs to be done on your own. Weight is never a group responsibility; it is an individual problem. But good luck, whatever route you go.

What about vitamins? There is great controversy in medical circles regarding the claims made by vitamin enthusiasts. At best, it must be acknowledged that for some people vitamins have had very positive effects. It can also be stated that taking vitamin or mineral preparations will not harm you.

Those who scoff at vitamins often dismiss them by saying, "It's all in your head; there is no scientific evidence to support the claims for them." Whether this is true or false is not nearly as important as the underlying assumption by which the efficacy of vitamins is being challenged. To say, "It's all in your head," is a serious miscalculation of the importance and power of the mind and emotions regarding overall fitness.

I have experienced freedom from all colds for more than four years. It was four years ago that I started taking a gram to 3 grams a day of vitamin C. Nothing else in my lifestyle changed. For me, therefore, vitamin C seems to have had a beneficial effect. I don't care if "it's all in my head," just so long as the cold isn't!

It is appropriate, while talking about diet and nutrition, to consider the American fascination with pills. In the consumption of drugs, we can see the American belief that for every ailment, need, and mood there is a pill to achieve the desired result. Fat people take pills to get thin, and many end up in worse condition than before they started. Some of the so-called diet wonder pills have been banned due to their adverse effect.

Pep pills are to be avoided, for pep (energy) should be the result of total fitness and cannot be successfully maintained through popping pills. Again, there are side effects which are very detrimental. Sometimes patients taking "mood elevators" forget when they were first prescribed. The doctor keeps filling and refilling the prescription. The patient increases the dosage, and a psychological addiction to the drug can take place. A person thus "captured" will often panic, with very unpleasant results.

One should be very cautious about developing a pill dependence as a permanent life-style, unless it has been professionally prescribed and the response to the drug is closely monitored by a physician. Many want to believe that for every personal distress there is a miracle drug, pill, capsule, or medication. Counselors frequently declare that what people really want is a shot of psychological penicillin. It does not exist. Let us accept this fact. Then we will be able to confront ourselves intelligently and manage our lives better.

Without any question, the most common addiction is smoking. There cannot be total fitness when smoking is involved. Smoking does not only damage the lungs; it decreases the oxygen-carrying capacity of red blood corpuscles, thus harming the entire body. It promotes heart disease, various respiratory diseases, cancer of all kinds, and early invalidism. It also makes one feel less well throughout each day of smoking.

On the opposite side of the ledger, there is not one good health reason for smoking. The notion that smoking keeps weight under control is not valid. Just for the fun of it, keep a mental record for a week or so of the number of people you see who do not have a weight problem yet who also smoke. You will be astounded to discover that very few of those who smoke are thin! Many who smoke compulsively also often eat compulsively. There is an excessive need for oral gratification that prompts smoking and eating. This behavior is prompted by the inability to handle tension in a healthful manner.

There are but a few people who maintain that they actually enjoy smoking. No amount of evidence for or against smoking moves them. There is nothing that I can tell you that you haven't heard before, and if you are going to smoke, it is your decision. If, however, functional fitness is to become your great priority, smoking will *not* be part of your new life-style. But, do not wait to stop smoking before starting to exercise.

There are dozens of methods for quitting. The success, however, lies not in the magic method but in the individual's total commitment to give it up. Although some will disagree, my personal belief is that if you are ready to quit smoking, you should tell no one. That's right, tell no one. Let your friends discover for themselves that you no longer smoke. You put an enormous amount of unnecessary pressure on yourself if you prematurely make public your resolution. Besides, it is *your* problem. You solve it, and let others make the discovery.

Perhaps sugarless gum will help; maybe drinking water, deep breathing, or just plain exercise will make it work for you. Individuals vary as to the aids employed, but those who want to quit must have an absolute commitment to quit. It's a small wonder that fitness is largely a question of psychology, will, and the ability to follow one's commitments.

As you approach the exercises in this manual, please bear in mind that total psychological commitment is necessary in order to achieve your goals. Physical fitness begins with a committed state of mind that governs your behavior every day in every way.

Posture

My father lived to be 90 years old, and he practiced medicine until he was 85. In fact, he made house calls after he was 80! Posture was a favorite subject of his. When his two oldest sons decided to become physicians, I can remember arguments about how to teach good posture. My father's prescription was the simplest and the shortest I ever heard. He simply said, "Stand tall." For whatever it's

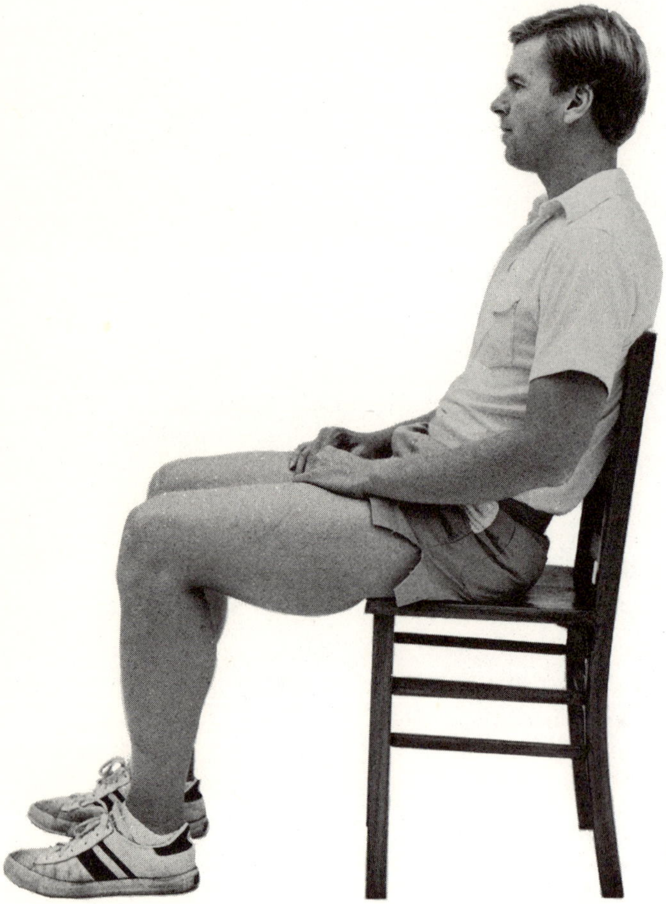

Don't sit like this. It's bad for the back, and tiring.

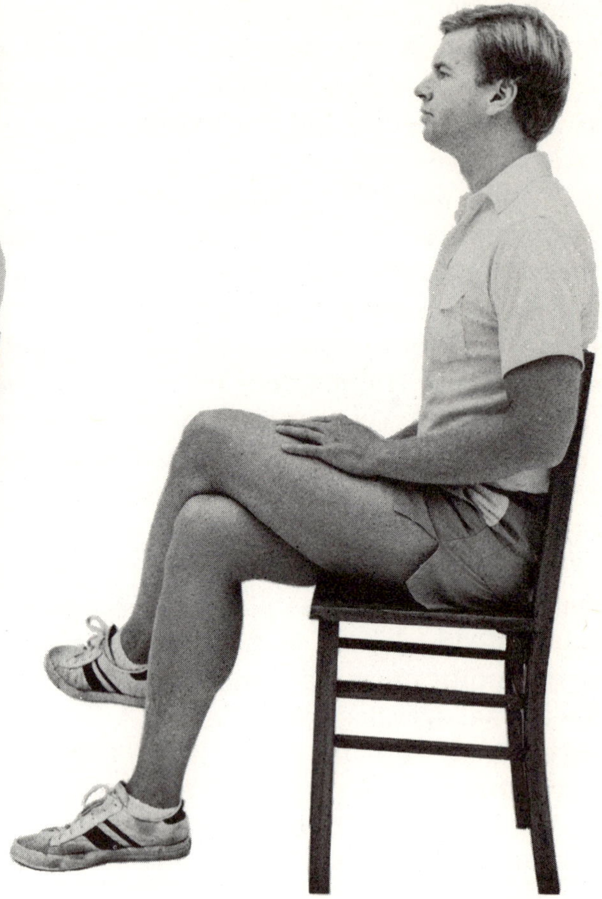

Do sit like this, back straight against back of the chair.

worth, that has worked for some people. Another old favorite is to stand flat against a wall, flat enough so that you feel your head and shoulders against it, and then step away from the wall while maintaining the same posture.

My own favorite is this one: Stand erect and extend your arms to the sides and at right angles to your body. Now, turn your palms up, facing the ceiling. Slowly lower your arms to your sides. When your arms touch your body, release your hands to their natural position. If this feels strained or tight through your shoulders, you probably have shoulder slump. Drooping shoulders produces stomach thrust; the center of gravity changes, and your body compensates in this manner. Stomach thrust puts additional pressure on the lower back which, in turn, causes backaches.

If you square your shoulders, stand tall, and have good abdominal tone, your posture will be good and your back will be less likely to ache. It is difficult for some people to accept the idea that good abdominal muscle tone has a direct bearing on the happiness and health of the lower back, but it most certainly does.

Posture while sitting is every bit as important as posture while standing. It may be even more important, because we often sit while working. Perhaps you have had the following experience: You sit in what appears to be a comfortable chair, and before you know it, you're sliding out. Avoid chairs that make it impossible for you to plant your feet (or one foot at least) on the floor while your back is touching the back of the chair. Most chairs have a back that is too short and a seat that is too deep. Sit in such a way that you can keep your back straight; one way to do this is to cross your legs, which braces your back against the back of the chair.

There is one simple solution to all problems of posture. We are actually not constructed to walk in an upright position. To relieve the pressure of gravity on your spinal column, get down on all fours (hands and feet, not hands and knees), and your back will feel great. However, your knuckles will get raw and you'll notice a lot of raised eyebrows, especially when you get on the bus! Short of getting down on all fours, you can follow the simple advice above and also wear good shoes that fit your feet. Good luck!

Protecting the Back

Most of us, sooner or later, end up with a back problem, and usually it's our own fault. In addition to performing regular exercises to strengthen muscles that support the back, you may need to change your ways of bending and lifting. Once these new methods become ingrained in your daily routine, an aching back is much less likely.

First of all, train yourself to reach with your legs. "Reach with my legs?" Yes, *with your legs.* To reach with your legs does not mean to stand on tiptoes. No, not that at all. It means that when you have to bend down, *bend your legs,* not your back.

The orthopedist often encounters a patient with severe pain in the lower back occasioned by nothing more than bending over the lavatory basin to splash water on his or her face. Why should such a simple movement as this result in such excruciating pain? The technical reasons are not worth detailing, so suffice it to say that when one bends at the waist with the legs straight, an unusual strain can be placed on the lower back.

It is unfortunate that plumbers and architects put sinks so low. Chances are you will not raise your sink, but you can lower your body by bending your knees while keeping your back reasonably straight. (Actually, the easiest way around this whole dilemma is to wait until you shower to get your face washed!) However, if you must bend down, let your legs do the bending. It will feel awkward at first, but

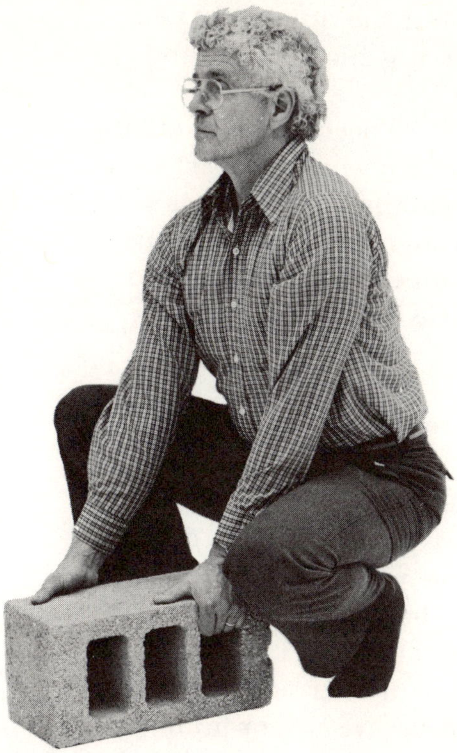

When you have to bend down or lift, bend your legs, not your back.

soon it will become a habit with you. The same principle can be applied to many other functions that you perform each day.

If your bath has a combination shower and tub, you must remember to bend with your legs to reach down to the faucets. (Why the faucets are always so low is another mystery of the trade.) If you must, *crouch* rather than bend at the waist in order to turn on the faucets.

Ordinarily, toweling off is hardly thought of as exercise. Done properly, it can reinforce your consciousness of keeping your back as straight as possible. While drying off, never let your profile be that of a hairpin! When it is time to dry the feet, sit on the john and bend only as much as you need to. Bring your foot up to you by placing it across your other leg. Obvious? Simple? Yes, but the number of people who hurt their backs by not observing such simple and obvious procedures is legion.

It may have occurred to you that I seem to be "coddling" the lower back. No orthopedic surgeon would suggest that these precautions are, in fact, "coddling." The back is extremely vulnerable to injury through carelessness, obesity, and performing simple tasks improperly. As you learn to depend on your arms and legs more, your back will ache less and you'll have more pep!

Knee Care

If the back is extremely vulnerable to accidental injury, the knees are not far behind. While we generally think of knee injuries as happening only to those who play football, basketball, or hockey, anyone can have badly sprained, twisted, or torn knees from other activities. The knee is a very special joint that requires careful attention. It must sustain tremendous impact whenever we run or jump. With each step the knee takes a stress of 3½ times body weight.

When we are young, the knee can take a lot of abuse. As we grow older, the joint often loosens, ligaments are stretched, and muscles not properly conditioned cannot keep the joint firm. Recently, I talked with a man who was recovering from an auto accident ten months before that produced fourteen fractures between his knee and his ankle. That is a lot of breakage. The exercises suggested to him are the same ones that I will recommend to you. The exercises in this book are remedial for those who require remediation. The same exercises for those without need of remediation should be viewed as a program of preventive maintenance.

How often, as a PE coach, I have heard a teenager boast, "I don't need any special knee exercises. My legs are terrific." A year or two later I would see the same young man, knee scarred by surgery, gingerly approaching the task of rebuilding the injured knee joint. In no way do I suggest that knee exercises can preclude all injuries for those in vigorous contact sports or skiing. What knee exercises can do, however, is *lessen* the possibility of injury, and for the nonathlete, they can ensure strong performance for years to come. This applies to the overwhelming majority of people, athletes and nonathletes alike!

"Fitness . . . is not something outside of you that you purchase or absorb; it is something inside. You must accept responsibility for your own health by utilizing the resources that are in you. They are there, ready to serve you if you will take the time, have the patience, and observe the regimens consistently."

Daily Exercises for Fitness

Warm Up or Loosen Up?

An age-old myth from traditional PE is the notion that an extensive warm-up period producing perspiration should precede physical exercise. Ask yourself why those stellar ballet dancers and gymnasts that you see on TV rarely seem to be exerting themselves. If they perspire at all, it is generally because of the bright lights and not because of their routines. Prior to the competition (or dance) you will observe the participants loosening up but not warming up. Functional fitness involves suppleness, and suppleness is derived from loosening up, stretching slowly and properly. This does not, of necessity, result in red cheeks or a wet sweatsuit.

Perspiration is an antiquated test of an individual's effort. Professional dancers, gymnasts, swimmers, and distance runners are among the very best-conditioned athletes in the world. If you observe them before their specialties, you will not see red-faced, puffing, sweating individuals. You will see people methodically stretching, deep breathing, and just generally limbering up.

Traditionally, perspiration has been viewed as the coach's measure of your effort, how hard you're "putting out." In this program *you* are your own coach. Measure your progress honestly, and you won't need to take a

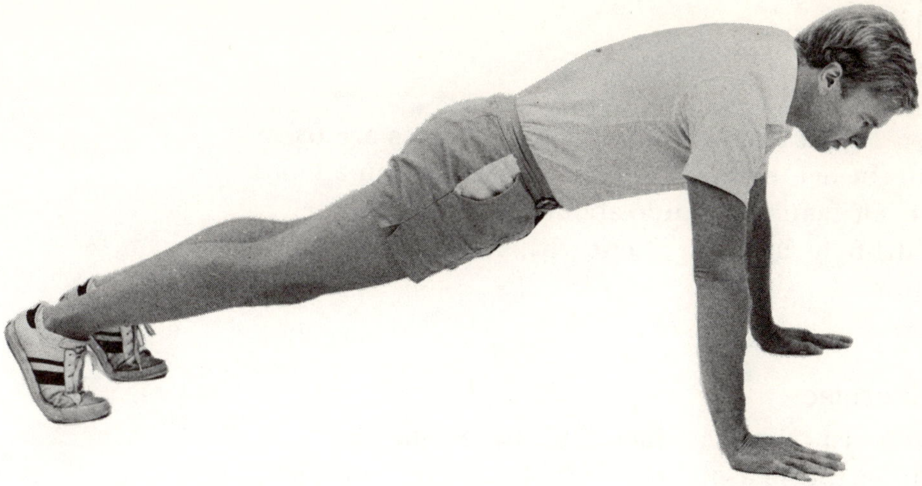

perspiration test. If fitness is viewed as stamina, strength, and suppleness, perspiration is not an objective or mark of accomplishment. You must ask yourself, "Am I more supple? Is my stamina increasing? Am I growing somewhat stronger?"

While we are talking about strength, let's puncture another illogical myth. Reasonable strength (for effective everyday functioning) will not result in ugly, bulging muscles. There's considerable evidence that bulging muscles and strength are not necessarily synonymous. You need not worry about gaining a muscular look because of having participated in this program.

Loosening up results from all of the exercises that involve stretching as opposed to those that are designed for strength. If the emphasis is on stretching rather than resistance of one muscle group opposing another (push-ups, sitbacks, neck pull), you are loosening up. Doing the exercises described will guarantee both loosening and strengthening. Do the routines in the order given, and you will build both suppleness and strength—to say nothing of increasing your stamina.

Keep uppermost in your thinking that FITness, not FEATness, is your goal. Fitness is the great feat to be achieved here. What feats accompany your fitness are truly secondary to the achievement of fitness itself. If you adopt a relaxed (but not casual) attitude about this program, observe it faithfully, and be patient with yourself, you can achieve fitness.

When to Exercise

People often insist that they "just don't have time to exercise." In part, this assertion stems from the traditional view of what constitutes exercise. One thinks of a special change of clothes, a gymnasium, other people involved in a game, or a group workout. Perhaps this is then followed by a steam bath, a swim, and a shower. Obviously, the better part of an hour or more is gone.

In our society, such time is just not available to millions of busy people. As a result, too many people will postpone their exercising to either a weekend activity or just before bedtime. Neither pattern is truly productive. First of all, those who reserve exercise for a weekend generally are involved in a competitive sport. While fitness is required for sports, most people want to believe that playing the game will result in fitness.

This is true, to a degree. The larger truth, though, is that one must have *overall fitness* to function each day in every way and not just for special expertise on the tennis court, the golf course, or the bowling alley. Of these three, only tennis (singles) can provide any meaningful cardiovascular exercise.

The best time to exercise is all the time. All the time? Yes, in the sense that virtually everything that you do every day can involve the principles underlying this program.

Naturally, it is best to devote a set amount of time each day to specific exercises. Although these can be done with benefit any time of the day, I believe that the very best time is first thing in the morning. This is likely to be the most convenient time, less likely to interfere with other plans, and can become as automatic as brushing your teeth. Exercises at this time take the stiffness and aches out of muscles and joints, limber you up, and prepare your body for the stresses and strains of the day to come.

Set your alarm 15 minutes early. Once you become familiar with the exercises in this chapter they can be performed in that amount of time. Do the exercises in the order shown each weekday (except those exercises marked intermediate or advanced; do only the exercises at your level). If you are running short of time, you may skip those exercises marked optional.

Strangely enough, you will require no extra room, equipment, or uniform. In fact, your pajamas are perfect garb. When the alarm sounds, turn it off and turn yourself on.

About the Exercises

If you have not been regularly engaged in an exercise program for some time, it is recommended that you follow the sequence of exercises straight through, but save the few exercises marked intermediate and advanced for later. Remember, it took you quite a while to get out of condition; it will require some faithfulness to get back into good condition.

Please, be patient with yourself. You are in competition with no one but yourself. Take each day's performance as it comes. Do not overdo. Doing too much too soon produces pain and stiffness, and this often forces a layoff for a few days. The days eventually become weeks, and all is forgotten.

Stick with it, and progress slowly. Advance to the next level only when you have mastered your current level.

Knee to Chest/Ear

(Stretching)

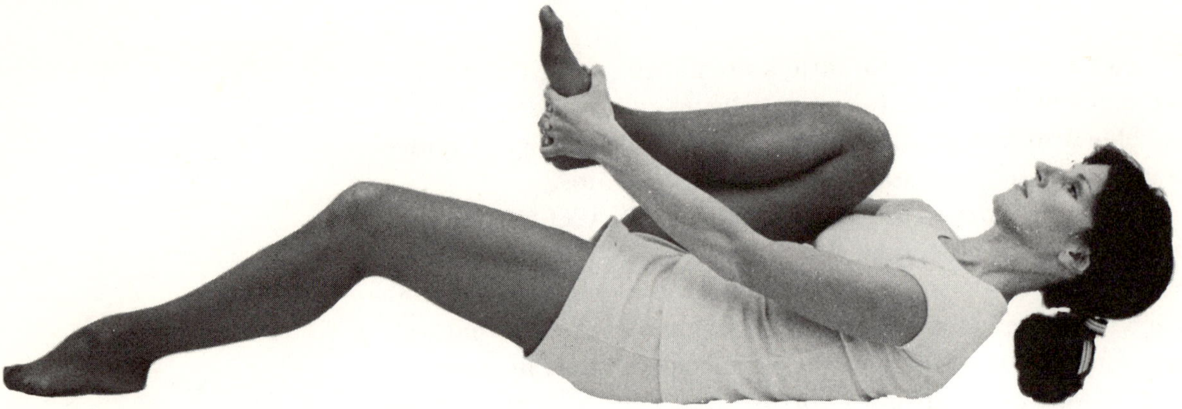

1 Using both hands, interlock fingers, reach down and grasp your heel (or knee, if you can't reach your heel), bringing knee slowly, firmly to your chest.

While lying in bed or on the floor with your knees bent, interlock your fingers and grasp your knee (or your heel, if you can), and pull your knee slowly but firmly to your chest. As you do so, curl forward with your body. Try to touch your right ear with your right knee, your left ear with your left knee. Do this 3 to 5 times with each leg, raising your body to meet your knee as you are drawing your knee to your chest. Next, clasp both knees, wrapping your arms around them, and curl up in a ball with both knees as close to your chin as possible. Hold this position for 15 seconds, then lie back and relax. You will never work up a sweat doing this exercise, but it has great value for the lower back. It will help to awaken you gradually and gracefully, and it also serves to loosen you up.

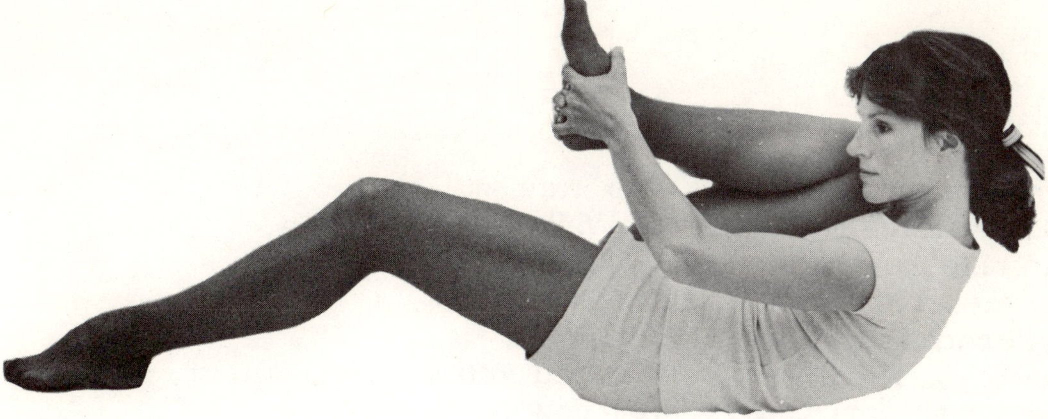

2 Curl upward and try to touch your right ear with right knee. Repeat exercise, touching left ear with left knee. Do both sides 2 or 3 times. Great for lower back!

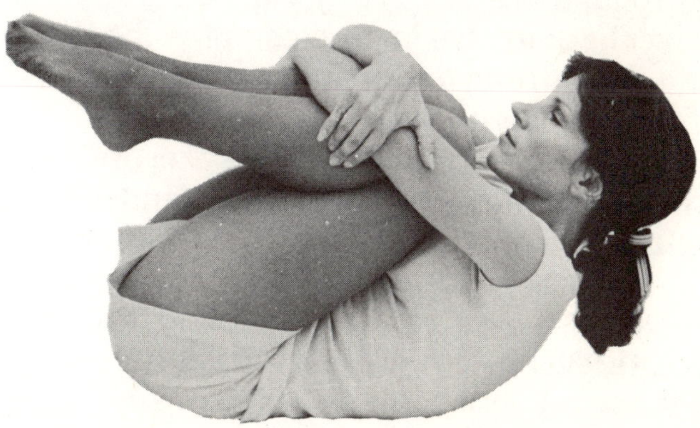

3 Clasp both knees, wrapping arms around them, and curl up in ball, knees to chin. Hold for 15 seconds, then lie back. This stretches lower back muscles, ligaments.

The Sitback

(Strengthening)

After you have finished the Knee-to-Chest exercise, sit on a carpeted floor for the Sitback exercise. While in a sitting position, raise your knees but keep your heels on the floor. Now, extend your arms straight in front of you and gradually lie back, keeping your back straight. Continue to lower yourself as if you were holding onto a bar with your extended arms. Lower yourself *slowly* after you are halfway lowered. Keep your back as straight as possible. You will be surprised at the amount of tension and stress you experience in the abdominal area. Going from 90 degrees to 45 degrees is fairly easy. It's the last 45 degrees that is the test. Go slowly! Finally, sit up, not too rapidly, resuming your original position. As you master this exercise you will want to increase the difficulty, as shown in the intermediate and advanced levels.

The stronger the abdominal region is, the less strain there is on the lower back. When your abdominal muscles are strong, there is no "belly sag." Belly sag forces the lower back to cave in, thus compressing the vertebrae and also putting undue strain on the muscles and ligaments of the lower back.

"But, how many times should I do this exercise?" Three repetitions are enough, if done slowly and with your back held as straight as possible throughout. It looks easy, but it is not. Be patient with your progress in this exercise. Do not move from the beginning level to the intermediate level (which will involve a different position for the arms) until it is truly easy to do 3 repetitions at the first level. If you find it very easy to do the beginning level from the very first time, chances are you are allowing your back to bend or you are moving too fast. Do the exercise honestly and it will help you—honestly!

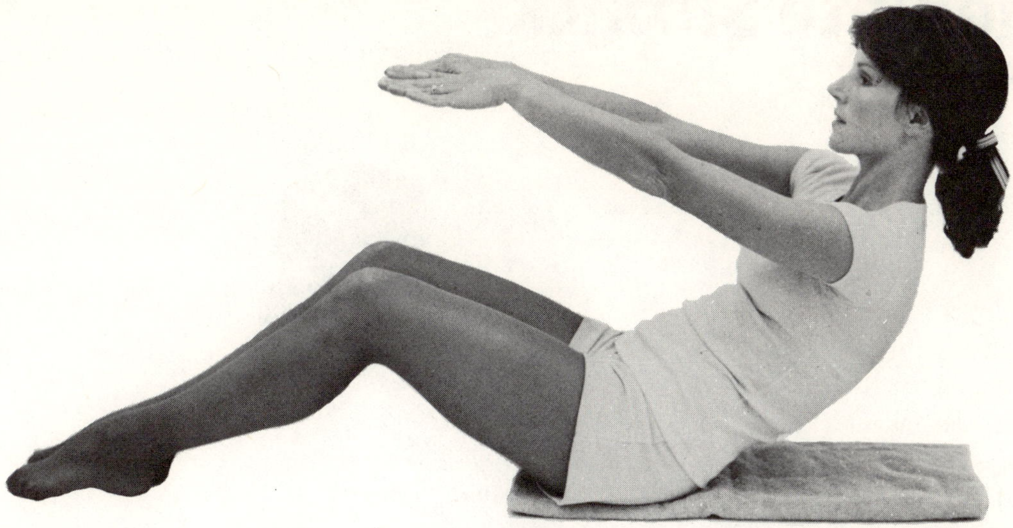

1 With arms outstretched in front, slowly lean back.

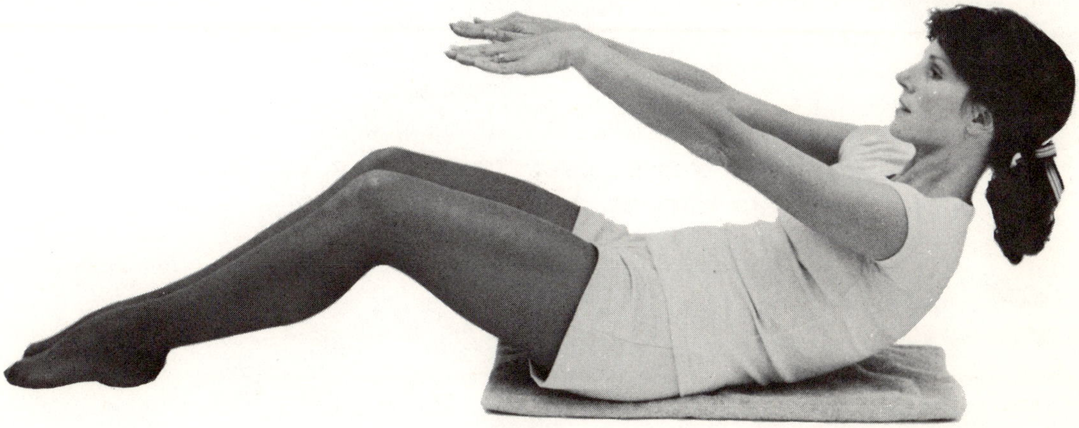

2 Lean back *very* slowly, keeping your back straight.

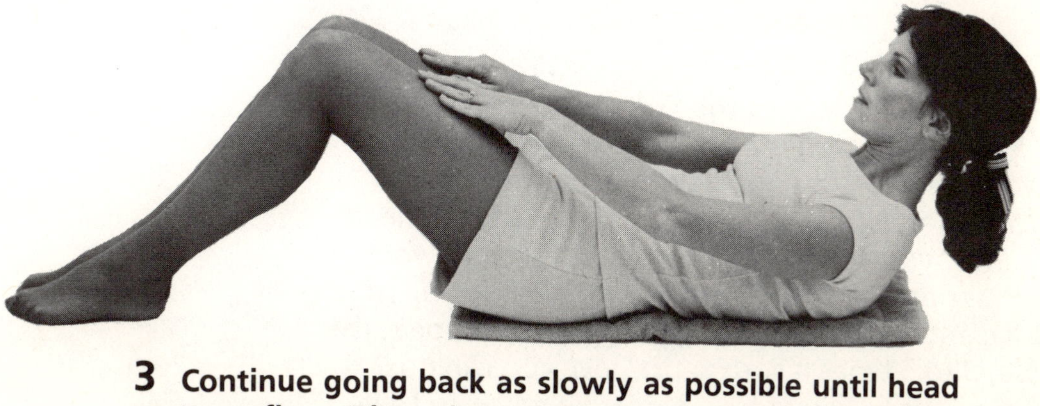

3 Continue going back as slowly as possible until head rests on floor. Then sit up, repeat exercise 3 to 5 times.

Intermediate Sitback

(Strengthening)

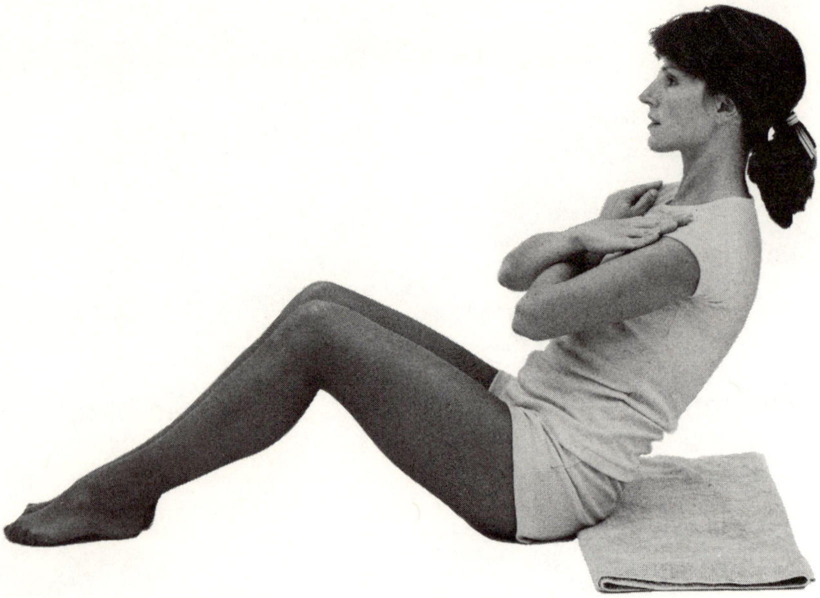

1 With arms crossed over chest, *slowly* lean back, keeping your back as straight as possible.

The Intermediate Sitback is the same exercise as the Beginner's Sitback, except the arms are crossed over the chest. While seated on the floor, raise your knees, but keep your heels on the floor. With your arms crossed over your chest and your back straight, gradually lie back. Lower yourself *slowly* until you are flat on your back, your head resting on the floor. Finally, sit up (not too fast), and resume your original position. Repeat the exercise; 3 to 5 times is sufficient. Once you can do 5 repetitions easily, you are ready for the advanced level.

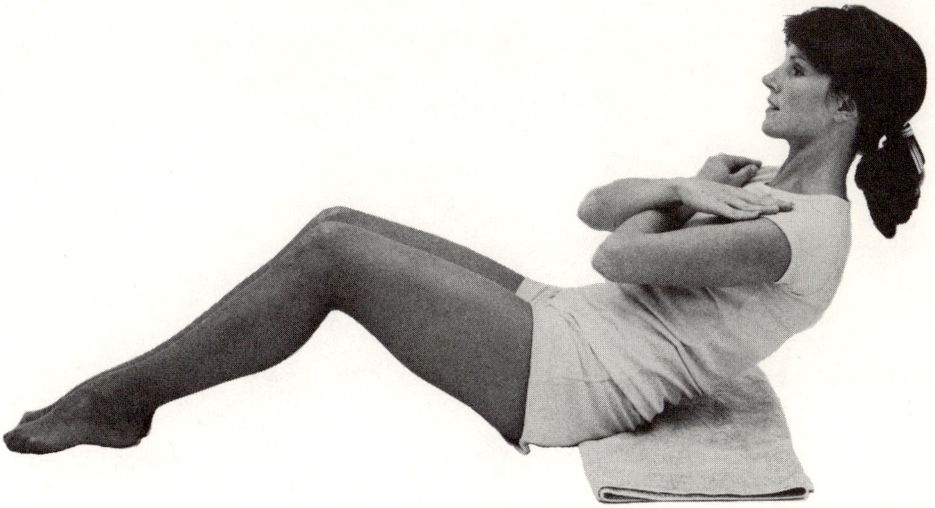

2 Keep leaning back, very slowly. Your back should be straighter than model's.

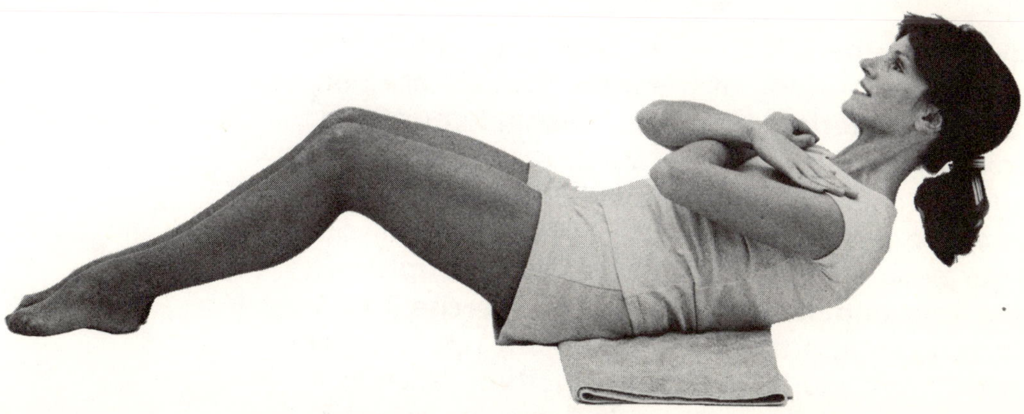

3 Lean back until your head is on the floor. Then sit up, repeat exercise 3 to 5 times.

Advanced Sitback

(Strengthening)

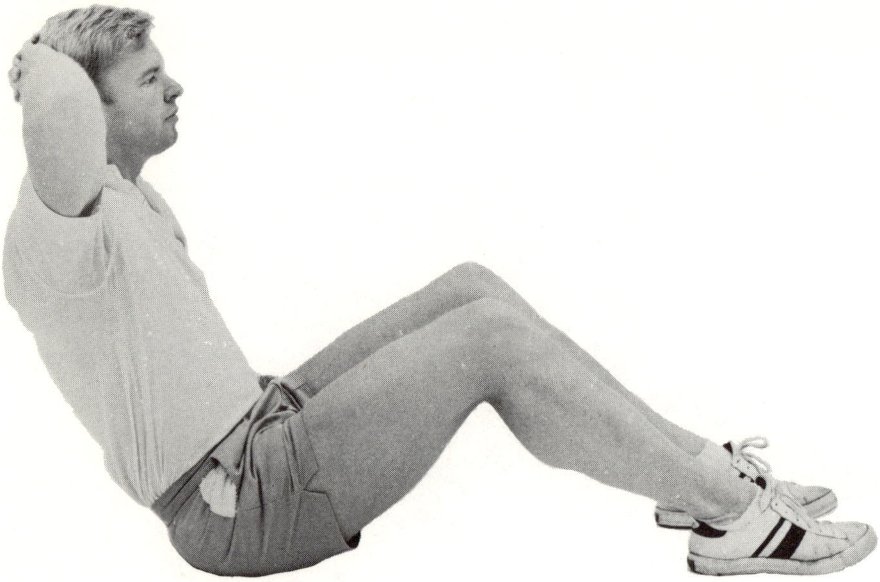

1 Interlock hands behind head, sit back *slowly*.

The Advanced Sitback is different from the others in just one respect: the position of the arms. While seated on a carpeted floor, interlock your hands behind your head. Raise your knees, but keep your heels on the floor. Keeping your back straight, gradually lie back. Continue to lower yourself *very slowly* until you are flat on your back, your head resting on the floor. Then sit up slowly, resuming your original position. Do the exercise 3 to 5 times. If you can't do the exercise without tipping over backwards, hook your toes under something, such as a couch. Try to employ your abdominal muscles as much as possible in the process, though, rather than relying on your leg muscles.

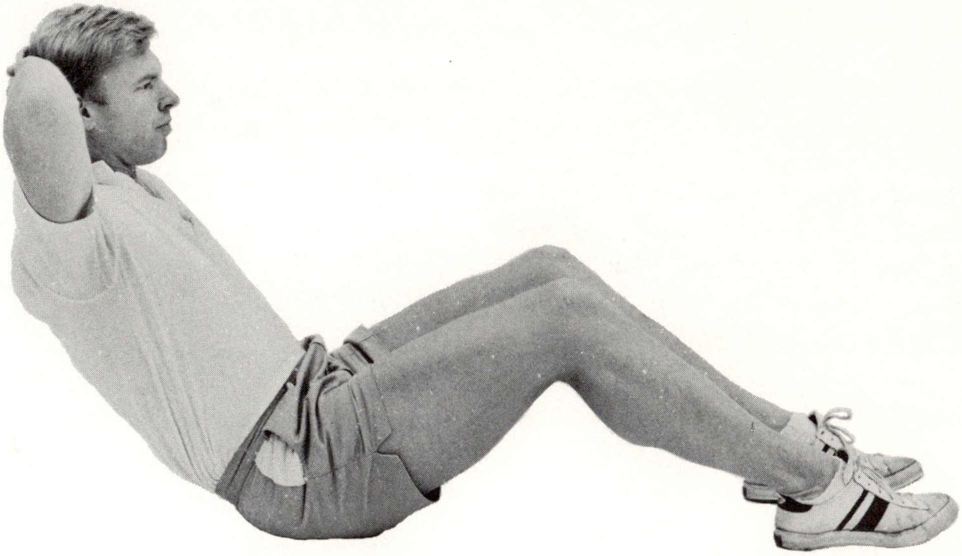

2 Gradually lean back, keeping your back straight.

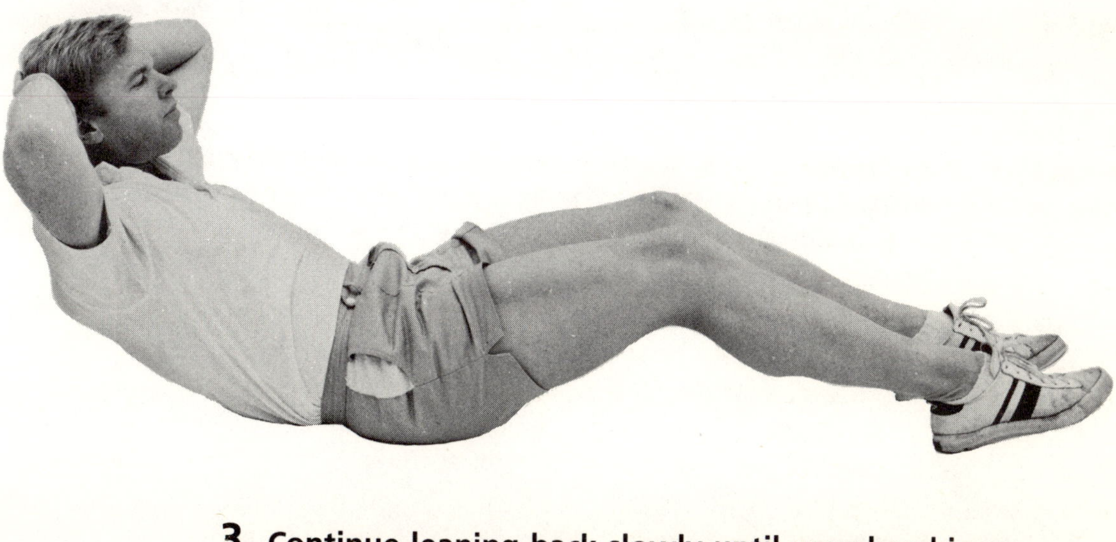

3 Continue leaning back slowly until your head is on floor. Then sit up, repeat exercise 3 to 5 times.

Supine Stretch
(Stretching)

Lie on your back. Try to touch the wall behind you with your hands and the opposite wall with your toes. Really stretch! Stay stretched out, back flat on the floor, for at least 10 to 15 seconds, then relax and breathe deeply. Repeat the exercise 2 or 3 times.

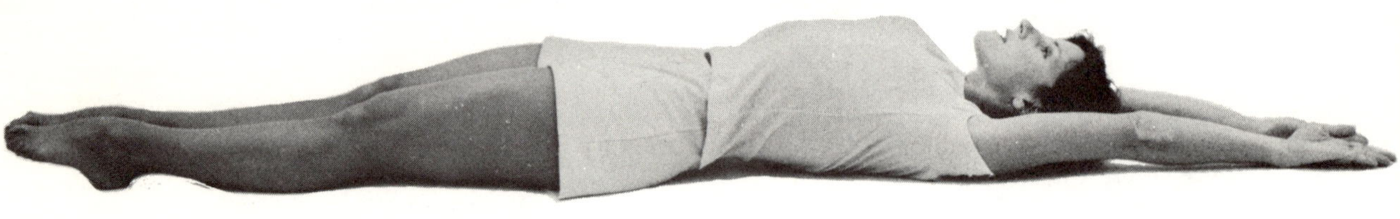

Flat on your back, try to touch wall behind you with hands, opposite wall with toes. Stay stretched out 10 to 15 seconds, then relax, breathe deeply. Repeat the exercise 2 to 3 times.

The Praying Press
(Strengthening)

For this exercise, which is done while standing up, put your hands together with your fingers extended straight up as if you are praying. Palms should be snug together, as should your fingers. Raise your elbows up so that your arms are nearly parallel to the floor. Now, just push and push and push for 30 seconds, as if you were trying to push your hands through each other, and then relax. You should feel this exercise in the upper chest or bust, particularly when you stop doing it. Its value is in firming the bust and the muscles of the upper chest. Do it 2 or 3 times.

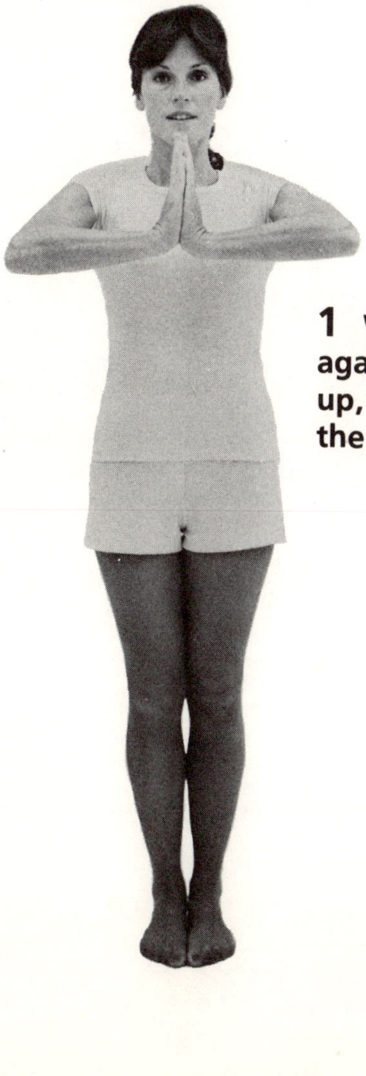

1 While standing, place hands flat against each other, fingers pointing up, your lower arms parallel with the floor.

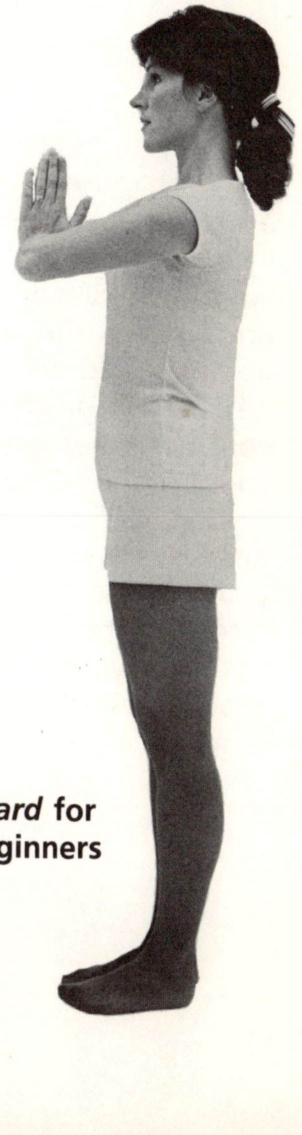

2 Press hands together *hard* for 30 seconds, then relax. Beginners do exercise 1 to 3 times.

The Neck Pull

(Strengthening and Loosening)

This is a good exercise for strengthening and relaxing the neck muscles (the area where tension headaches originate). While seated with your back straight, interlock your fingers and hands high on the back of your head. Slowly but steadily pull forward with your arms, but at the same time stiffen your neck so as to defeat the forward pull. Maintain this pressure between neck and hands for about 30 seconds. Relax by removing your hands, dropping them to your side, and allowing your head to drop down. Repeat the exercise 2 times. Try to touch your chin to your body. Do not rotate your head; just use an up-and-down movement. Rotating your head in broad circles can have a bad grinding effect on the disks between your vertebrae. It will also not do any more for your neck muscles than the procedure just outlined.

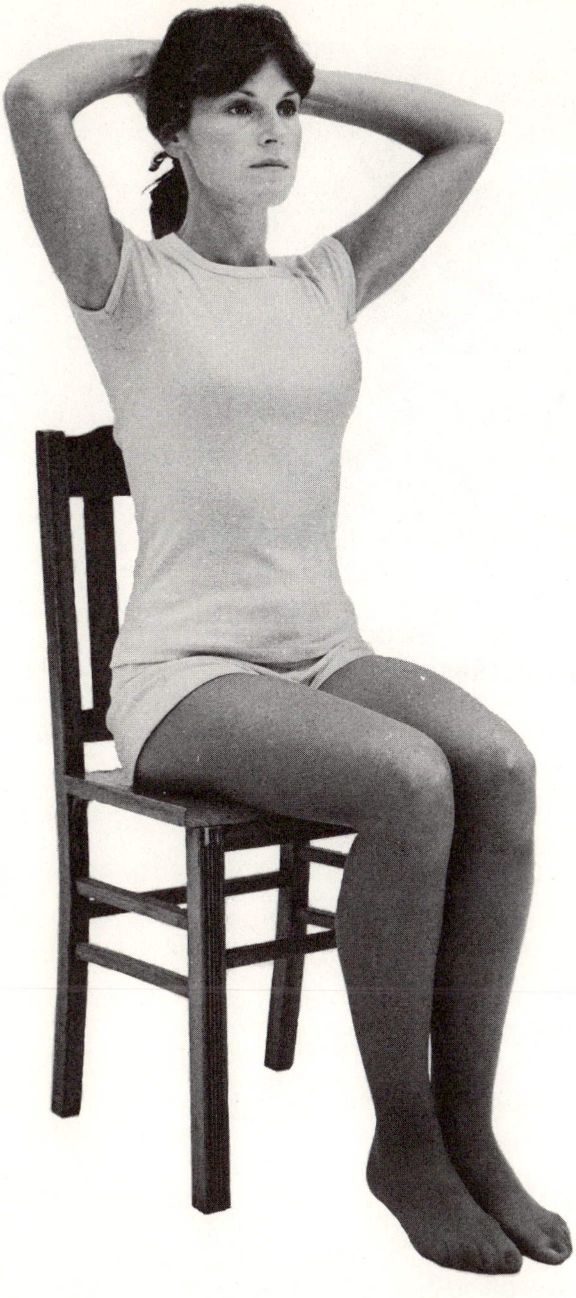

1 Sit erect, hands interlocked high on back of head. Stiffen neck, preparing for neck vs. arms tug-of-war.

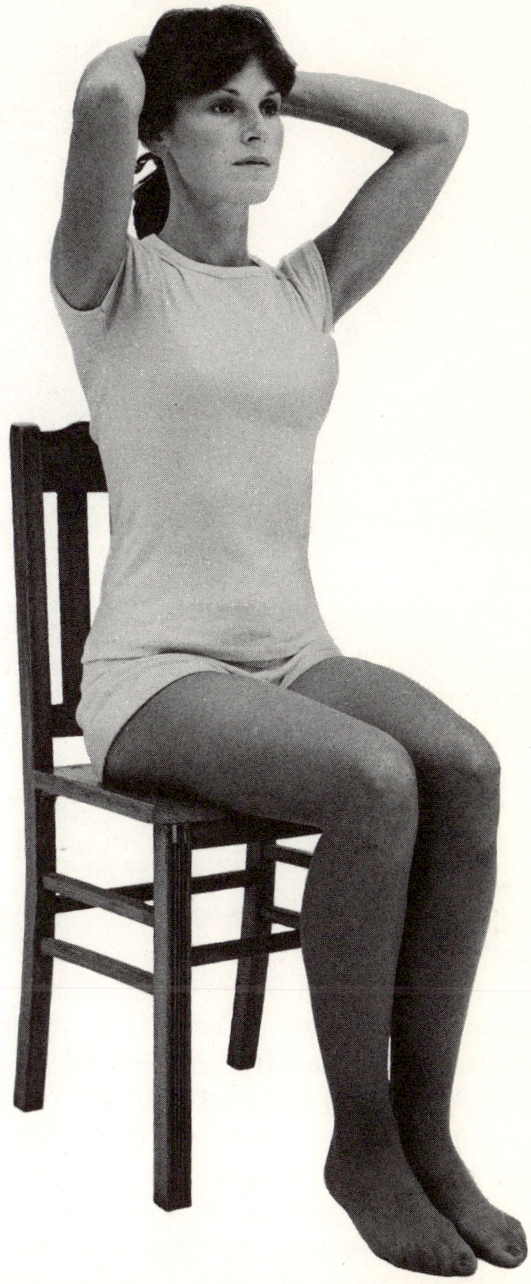

2 Slowly but steadily pull forward with arms while pushing back with head. Hold for about 30 seconds, then relax.

Gathering Marbles

(Strengthening) Optional

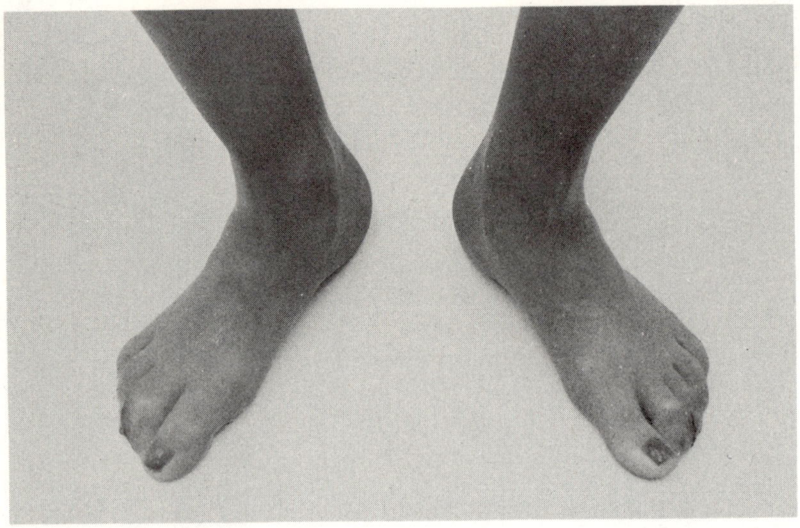

1 While seated on edge of bed, feet on floor, contract toes as if trying to pick up marbles.

The following exercise is very good for the feet and ankles, which are often neglected. While seated on a chair or edge of the bed with your feet on the floor, pretend that you are going to pick up marbles with your toes. Use a gathering and sweeping motion with both feet, while pivoting your ankles, as if you are trying to pile all the marbles together. You will discover quickly that this is a rather tiring exercise. After a minute or so of "marble picking," proceed to the next exercise.

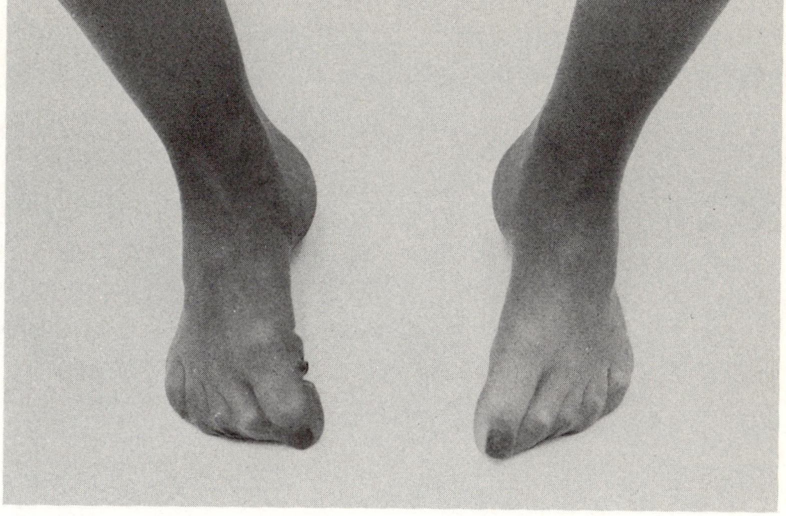

2 As you "pick up marbles" with toes, sweep feet together as if gathering marbles between.

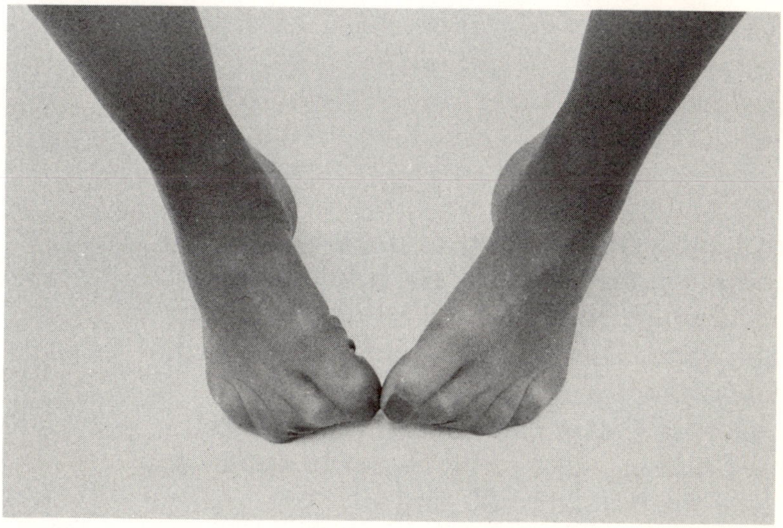

3 This is the final position. Repeat exercise 10 to 20 times. It not only limbers up ankles and toes but relieves aching arches and tired feet.

Crumpling Newspaper

(Strengthening) Optional

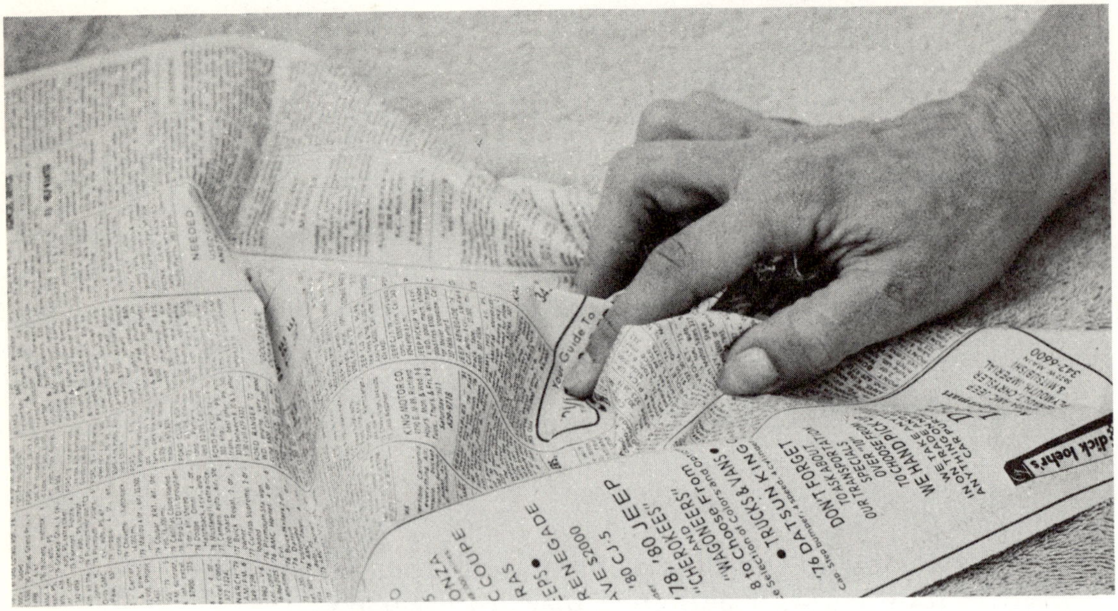

1 Take one full sheet of newspaper. Grasp one corner.

An excellent hand-strengthening exercise is available to anyone who gets a daily paper. Take a full sheet of newspaper and grasp one corner. Gather it into a ball, using just one hand. This exercise will feel awkward at first, but after a few tries it is simple to do. An alternative exercise that is even better is to grasp an ordinary small rubber ball or a worn-out handball and simply squeeze the ball 20 to 40 times.

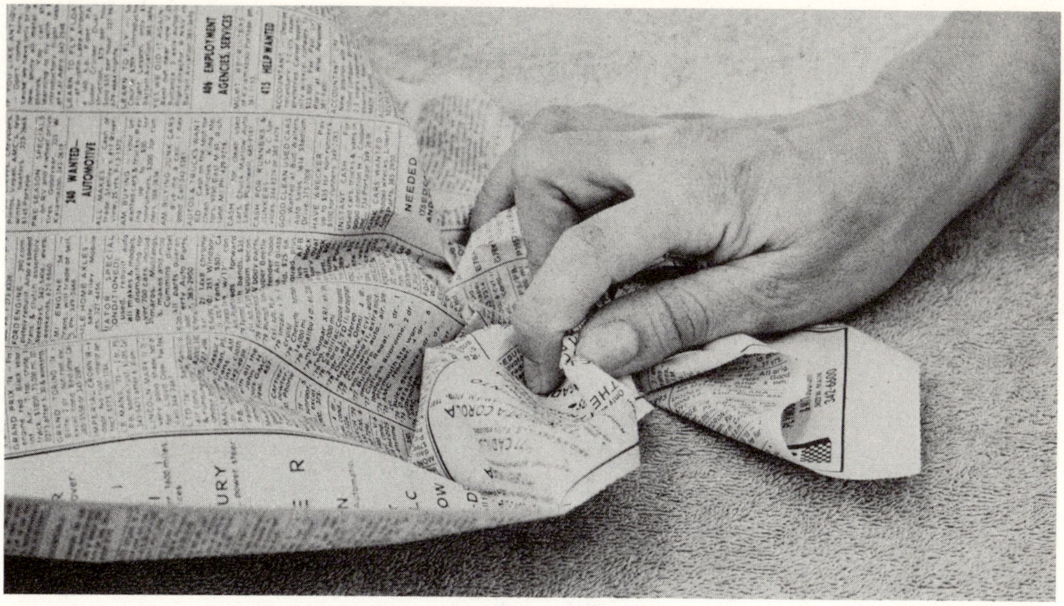

2 Start crumpling and gathering it into your hand.

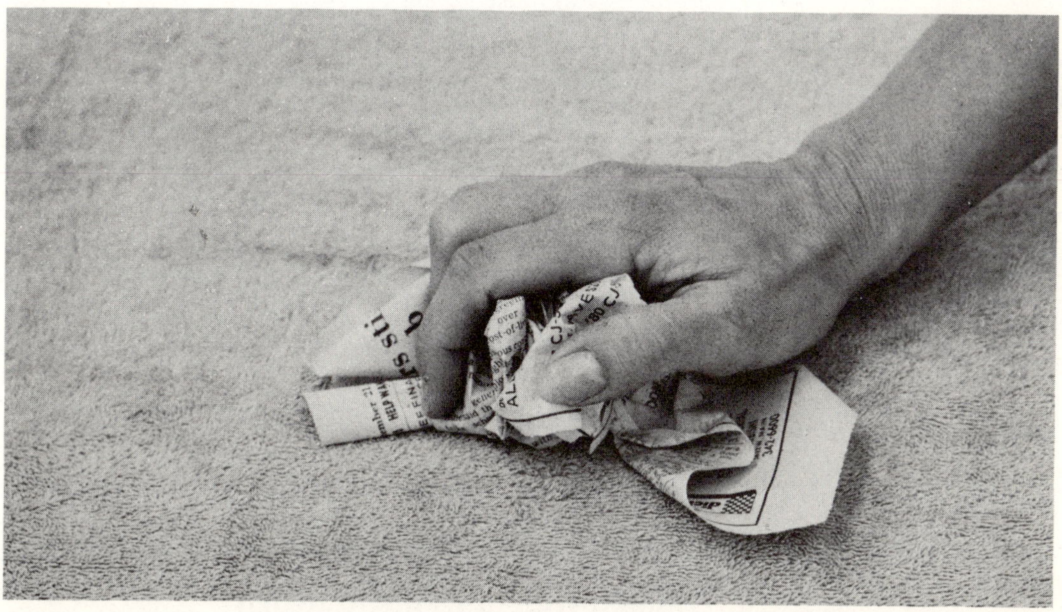

3 Crumple the entire sheet of newspaper into a ball.

The Bear Hug

(Strengthening)
Optional

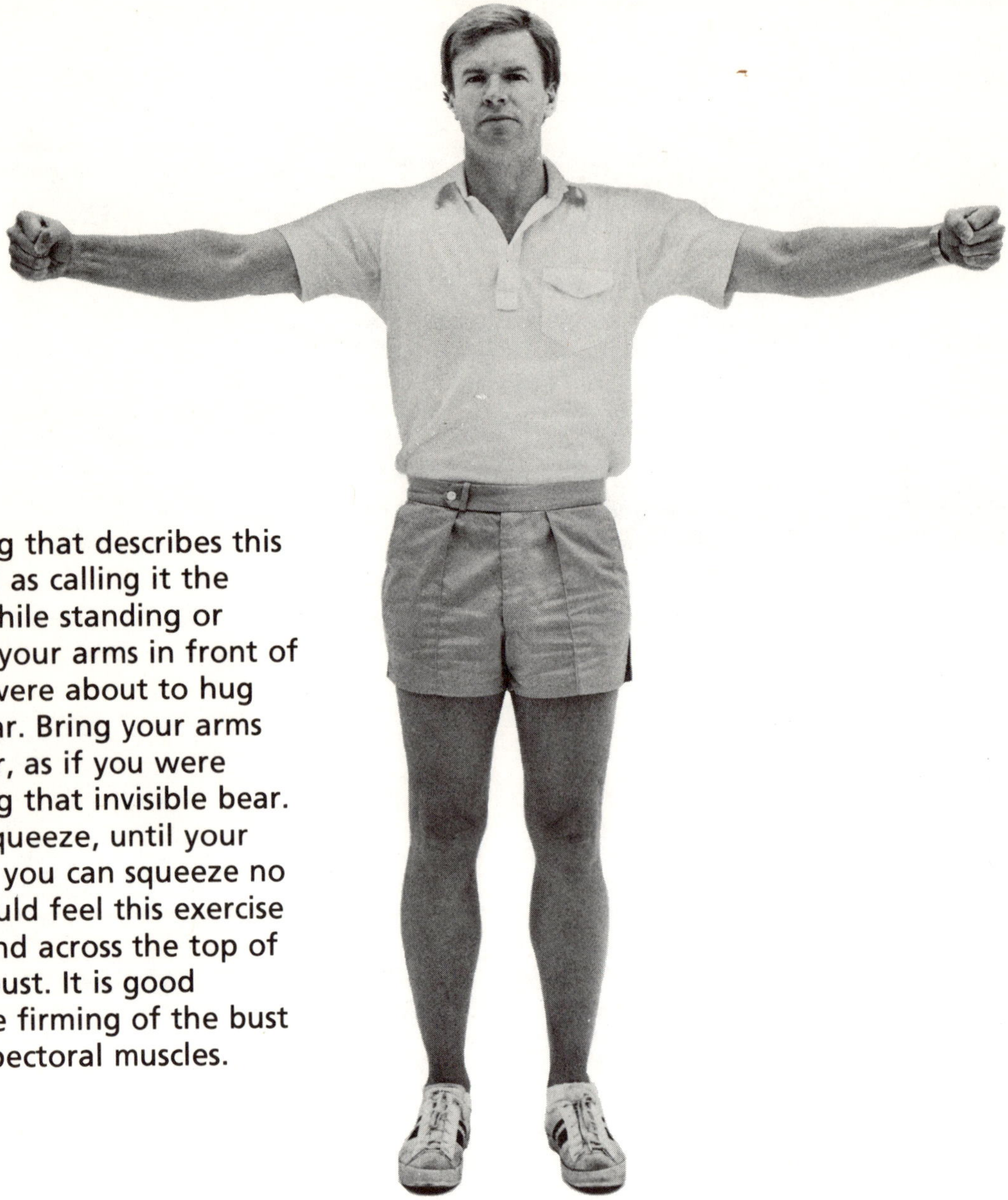

There is nothing that describes this exercise as well as calling it the "Bear Hug." While standing or sitting, extend your arms in front of you, as if you were about to hug an invisible bear. Bring your arms slowly together, as if you were really squeezing that invisible bear. Squeeze and squeeze, until your arms cross and you can squeeze no more. You should feel this exercise in your arms and across the top of your chest or bust. It is good exercise for the firming of the bust and the male pectoral muscles.

1 Begin with arms outstretched and fists clenched.

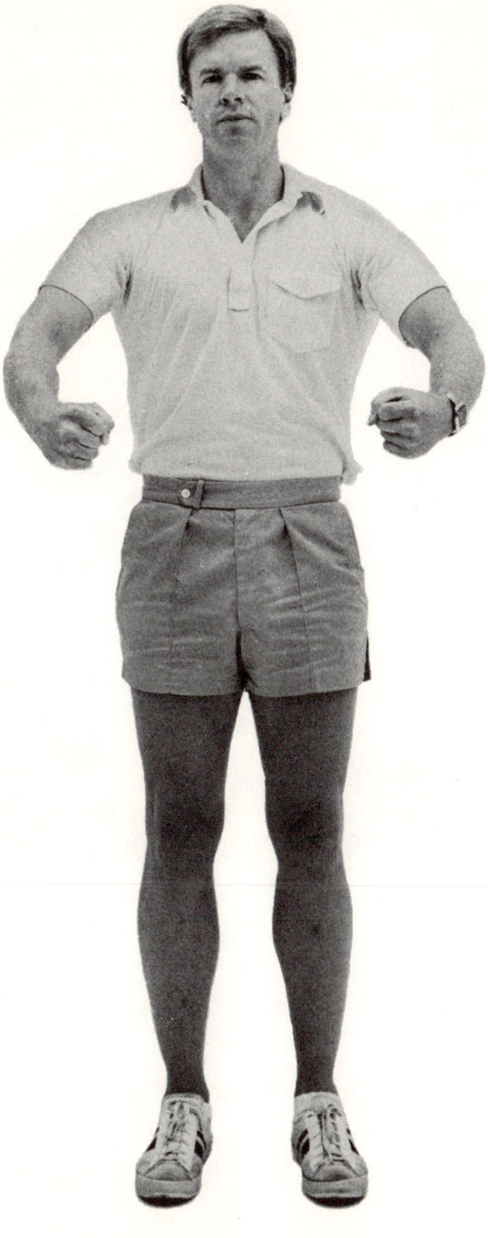

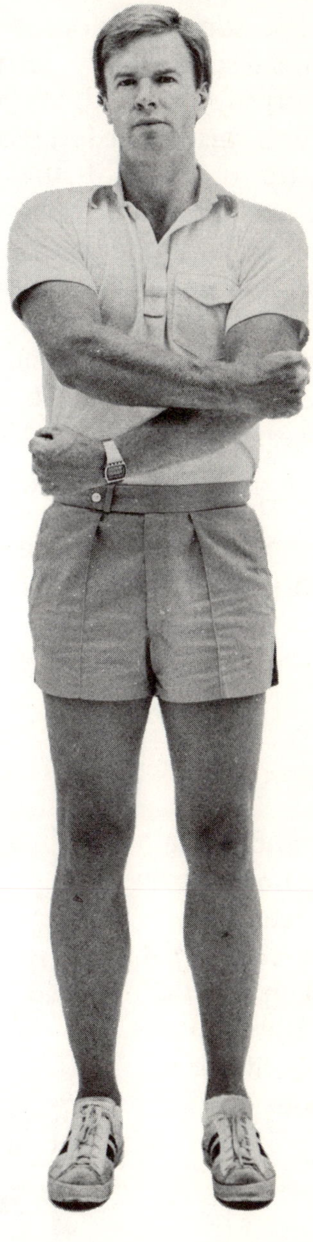

2 Bring your tensed arms together, as if hugging an invisible bear.

3 Keep squeezing, even after your arms cross.

Dancer's Exercise

(Stretching)

This is the recommended exercise to replace all forms of toe touching. Use some caution on this exercise, or you may fall down. Select a steady, large chair, a low dresser, or the footboard of your bed. Stand close enough to it so that when you raise your leg, you can rest your heel (toes pointing up) on the flat surface. Your raised leg should be straight. Once you have mastered the exercise your leg should be at 90 degrees to your body. The average person will have to start out at a lesser angle. If your raised leg will not lie straight, this tells you how tight and short your hamstring muscle is. Gently but firmly press down on the knee to straighten the leg. Release and press down at least 10 times. Eventually, after a week or two of daily exercises, the leg will straighten out. Then proceed to increase the stretching of the hamstring, as shown in the pictures. You can accomplish more stretching by raising the leg higher.

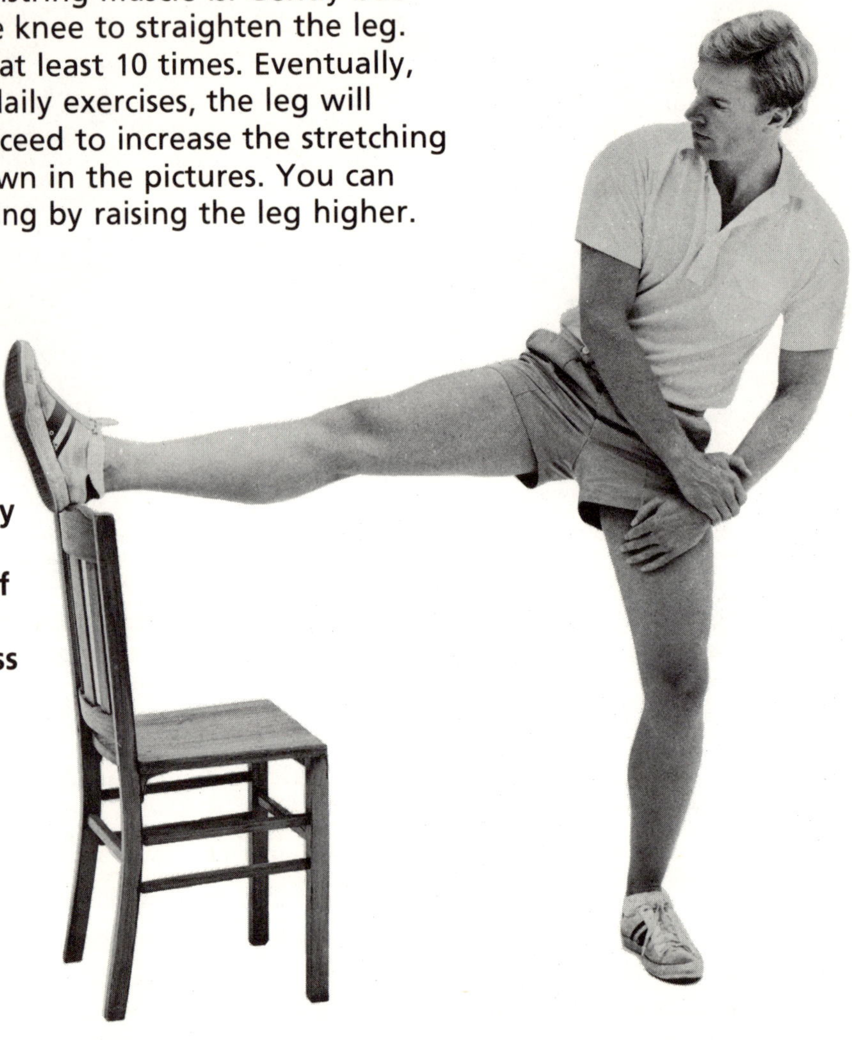

1 Raise leg and place heel (toes up) on sturdy support. Be ready to grasp nearby support if you teeter. Leg should be straight. If not, press down on it gently but firmly 10 times.

You should also "flex" the leg you are standing on (bend at the knee slowly) to increase the pressure on the extended, supported leg. Be sure that the toes of the extended leg are always pointing up and not pointing to either side. The raised foot must be vertical. This exercise should be done for both legs. Plan to spend at least 30 seconds with each leg each time.

Some people may find it difficult to maintain their balance while standing thus on one leg. Move the chair next to the wall, and you can catch yourself if you feel insecure or if you start to lose your balance. Do not attempt to raise your leg more than 90 degrees before you have the necessary suppleness. This generally results in a loss of balance. Be patient with your progress, but work at this exercise each day. Eventually, you may be able to raise your leg to shoulder height—not just 90 degrees.

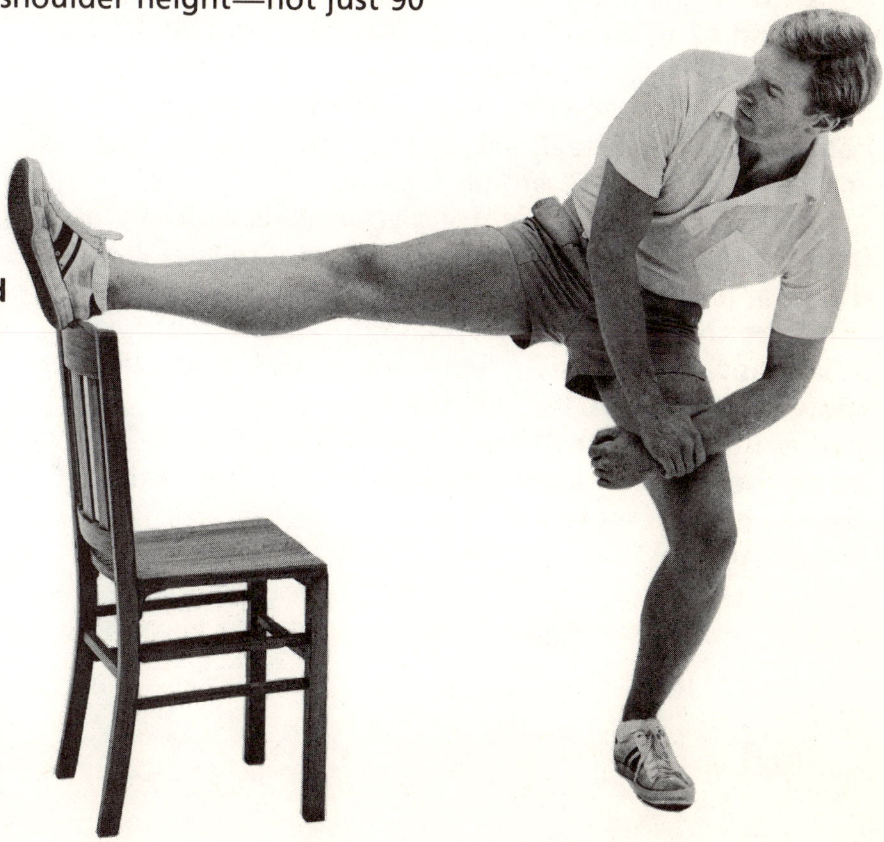

2 Eventually you should be able to raise leg until it is at right angle to body or higher. Bend standing leg in order to increase pressure on extended leg. Spend 30 seconds on each leg.

Toe-Ups

(Strengthening)

1 Shoes off, stand with toes and balls of feet on edge of plank, heels on floor.

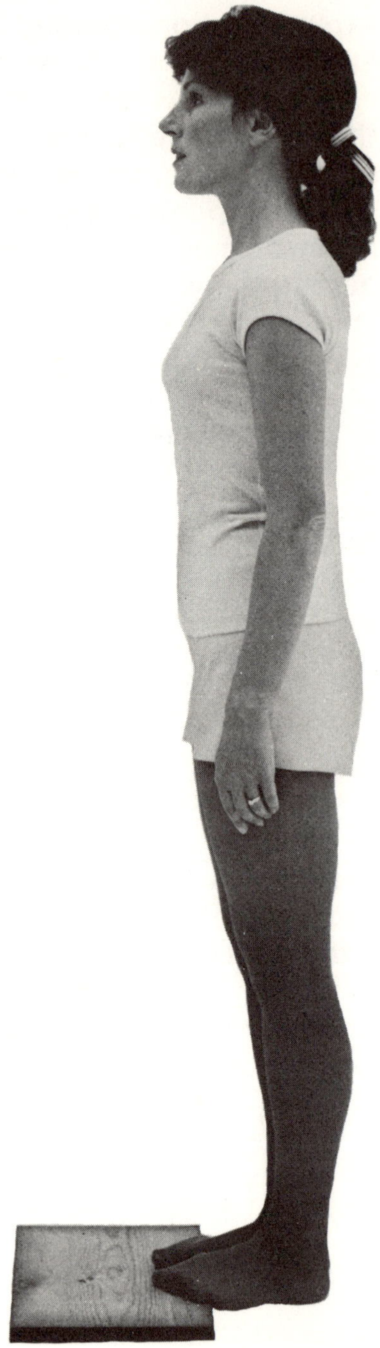

This is an excellent exercise for the calf of the leg and is good for the feet and ankles as well. You'll need a large book or a short plank about 2 inches thick, 8 inches wide, and 12 to 24 inches long. A book about the size of an "Annual" from an encyclopedia will do nicely. Place the book or plank on the floor. Put both feet on the book so that your heels are on the floor and the toes and balls of your feet are on the book. Now raise yourself up on your toes, lifting your heels well off the floor. Up and down, up and down. If you're shaky, do this in a doorway and steady yourself by placing your hands on the door frame. Up and down, up and down. How many times? They're your calves, and they'll let you know soon enough. But you ought to be able to increase the number of repetitions after a few days of doing toe-ups. Some people can start with ten; others may wish to try more.

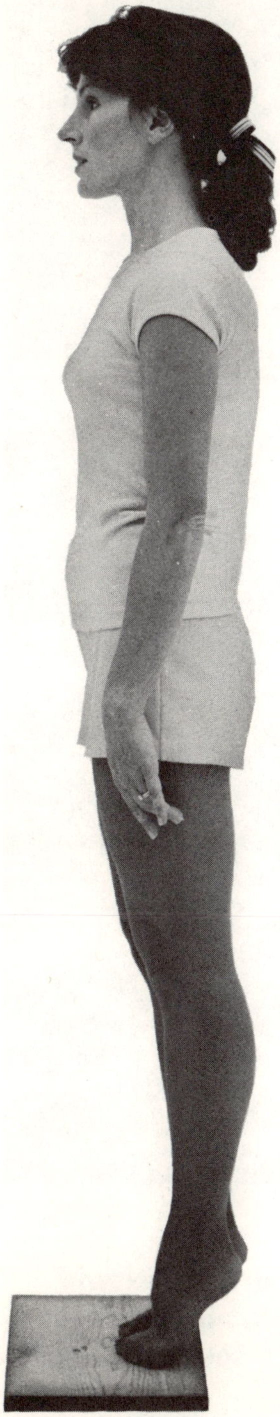

2 **Rise up on your toes, then down again—10 times or more—good for calf, ankles, feet.**

Arm Circles

(Stretching) Optional

Arm circles (not illustrated) are virtually self-explanatory. Extend your arms out to your sides with your palms down. Straighten and stiffen your arms, and make slow but pronounced circles. You should feel this in your upper back and shoulder. If not, bring your arms back and exert a little more "oomph" as you make the circles. Rotate forward and then backward in full-circle motion. You should do this exercise for at least 30 seconds. As you progress, you should increase the time to 60 seconds or even more. If you like, open and close your hands while doing the exercise. This gives it an added dimension which strengthens your hands and wrists.

Doorway Press

(Strengthening)

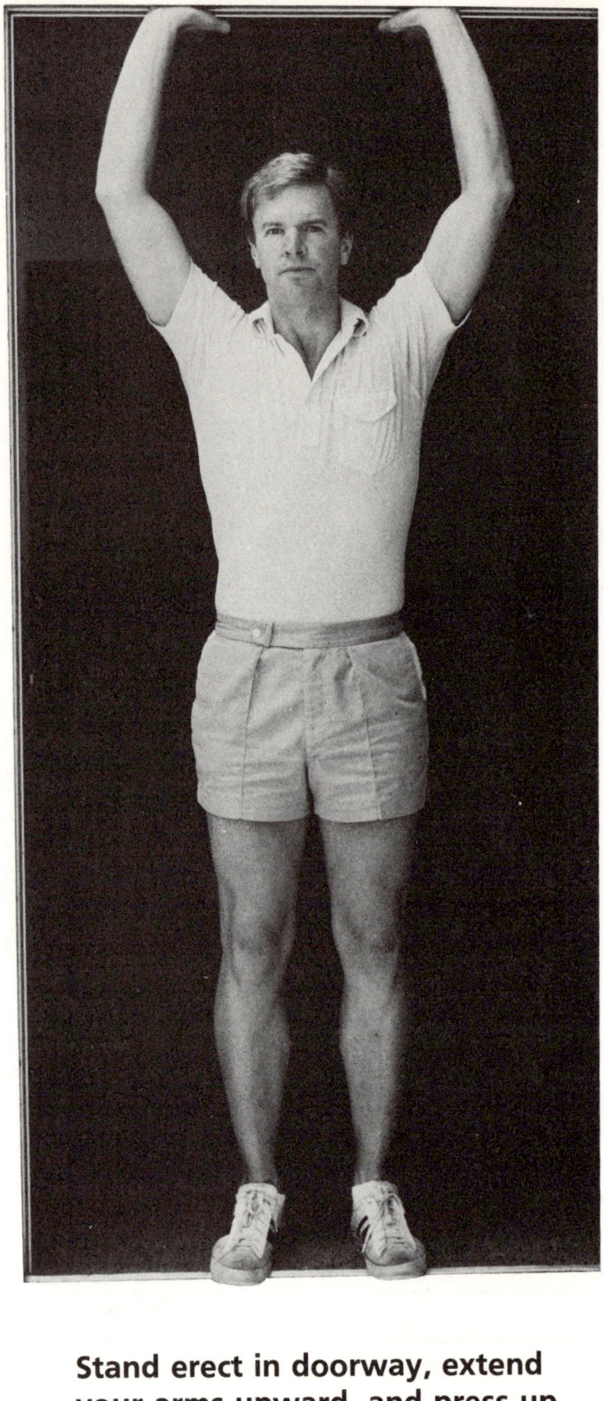

Proceed to a nearby doorway. Stand directly in the doorway. Extend your arms upward, placing your hands on the top of the door frame. Pretend that you are going to push the top of the doorway to the ceiling. Be sure you stand straight. Press slowly but with genuine effort for at least 5 seconds. Release, relax, and repeat 2 or 3 times. If you are too short (or the doorway is too high) to reach the area to be pressed upward, find something stable to stand on to do the exercise. Bend the knees, if necessary, but keep the back straight.

Stand erect in doorway, extend your arms upward, and press up *hard* for at least 5 seconds. Repeat 2 to 3 times.

Wall Sit

(Muscle Toning) Optional

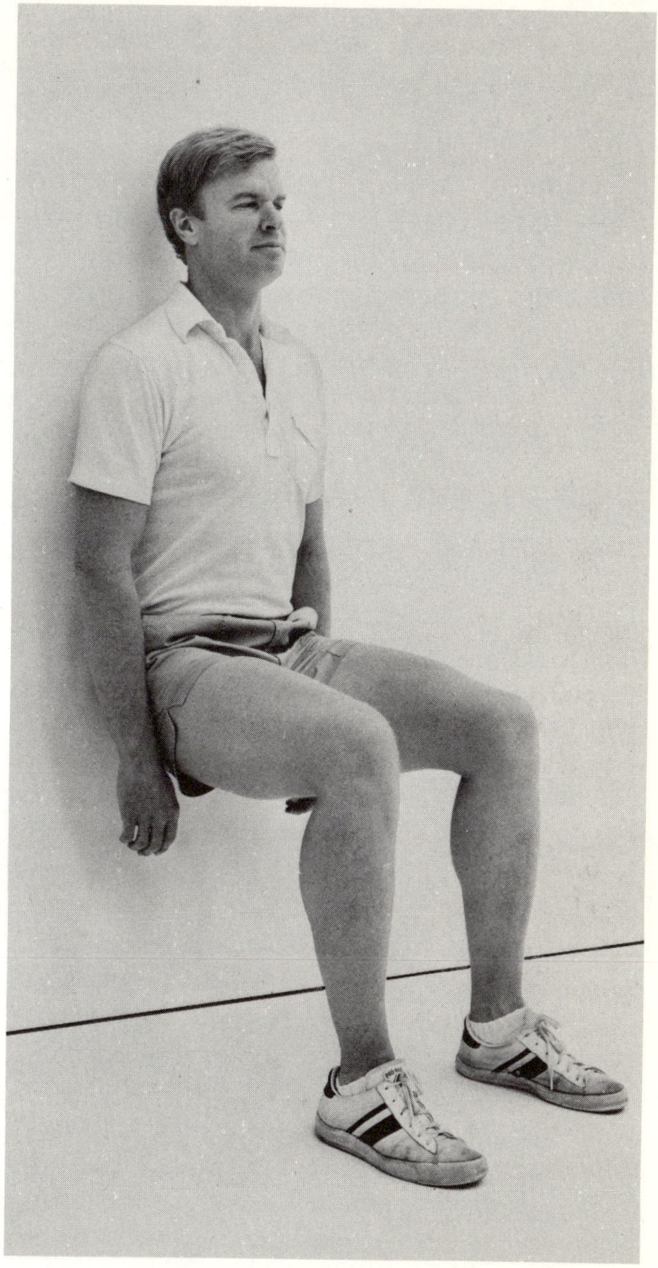

Sit "on air" with back flat against wall, head erect, legs making a right angle. Count to 20; each day increase the count.

If you cannot get into the bathroom yet, occupy your waiting time with yet another exercise. Of all the exercises in this program, this one appears to be the easiest. Assume a sitting position with your back against a wall. Simple, isn't it? Be sure that your feet are securely planted. Note that there is a right angle between back and thigh and between thigh and lower leg. These two right angles are very important in doing this exercise. Observe that the hands and arms hang loose at the sides, thus offering support. What do you do now that you've assumed this position? Just hold it for as long as you can, perhaps 15, 30, or 60 seconds. If you are a prodigious walker, you will find this fairly easy. If you are an average walker, your thigh muscles will soon sing out their complaint to you.

The Wall Sit is a very deceptive exercise. It looks incredibly simple, but in reality it is very taxing for most people. It is an excellent toning exercise for the thighs. Be sure that you keep the small of your back straight and flush against the wall and your head erect throughout this exercise.

Push-Ups
(Strengthening)

It is time for a few push-ups, which provide excellent exercise for the arms, shoulders, and upper back. On the following pages, you are given a choice to help you select the type of push-up most suited to you. Do not be discouraged if you must start with the beginner's position (knees to hands). This is suitable not only for beginners but for those who are overweight.

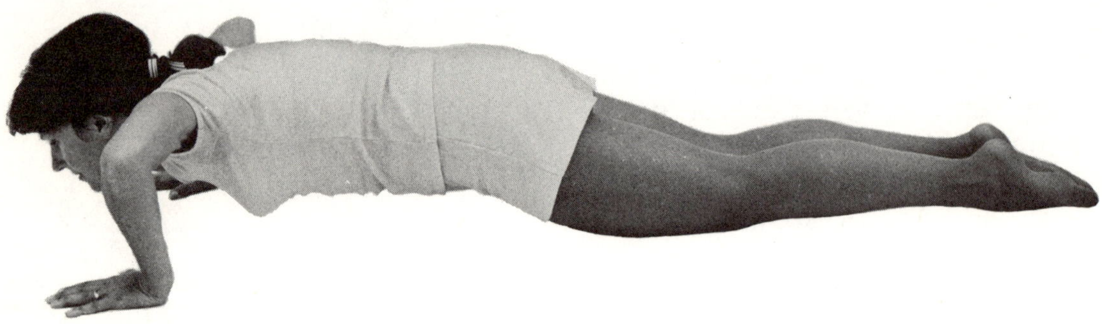

1 Begin lying face down on floor, hands flat with thumb of either hand directly beneath edge of shoulder. Keep back straight as you press away from the floor.

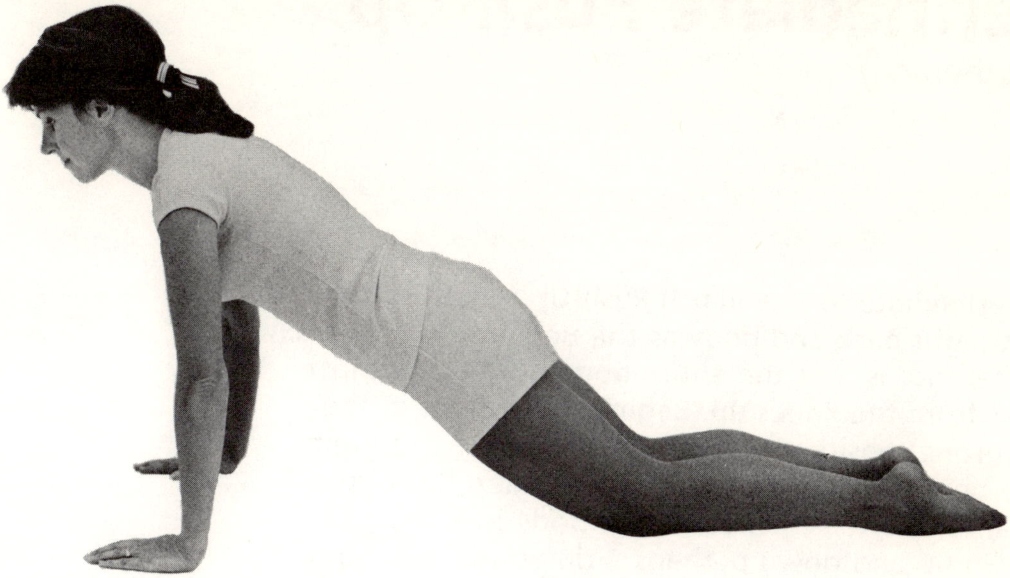

2 Press until arms are straight. Knees remain on floor. Now lower upper trunk until chest nearly touches floor and rise again, repeating exercise at least 2 to 4 times.

Beginner's Push-Up

(Strengthening)

Begin on the floor, in the down (prone) position, hands flat on the floor and positioned so that the thumb on either hand rests directly beneath the edge of each shoulder. This positioning is very important in order to give you maximum lift. Rest your knees on the floor, but keep your upper legs and trunk in a straight line throughout the exercise. Do not curl up or down.

Now straighten your arms, raising your body up, lowering it again until your chest nearly touches the floor. Go up, down, up, down, 3, 5, 7 or more times, but *do not rest your body on the floor* until you have finished the entire set of push-ups.

Intermediate Push-Up

(Strengthening)

The Intermediate (or standard) Push-Up requires the same straight back and body as the Beginner's Push-Up. The difference is that the entire body is lifted, not just the part from the knees up. Begin on the floor in the down (prone) position, hands on the floor with thumbs directly beneath the edge of each shoulder. Push up off your hands and toes, keeping your body in a straight plane. Go up and down perhaps 5 times, not touching the floor until you rest at the end of a set. When you have more practice, try for 10 push-ups in a set. Several sets like these, with rests between, are better than one extended set.

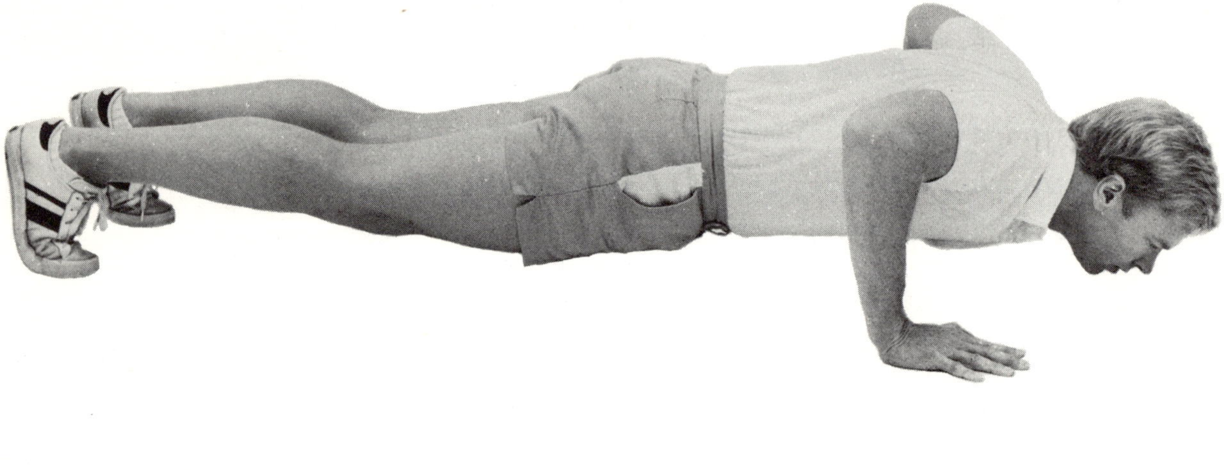

1 Begin lying face down on floor, hands flat with thumb of either hand directly beneath edge of shoulder. Push up off hands and toes, keeping body straight.

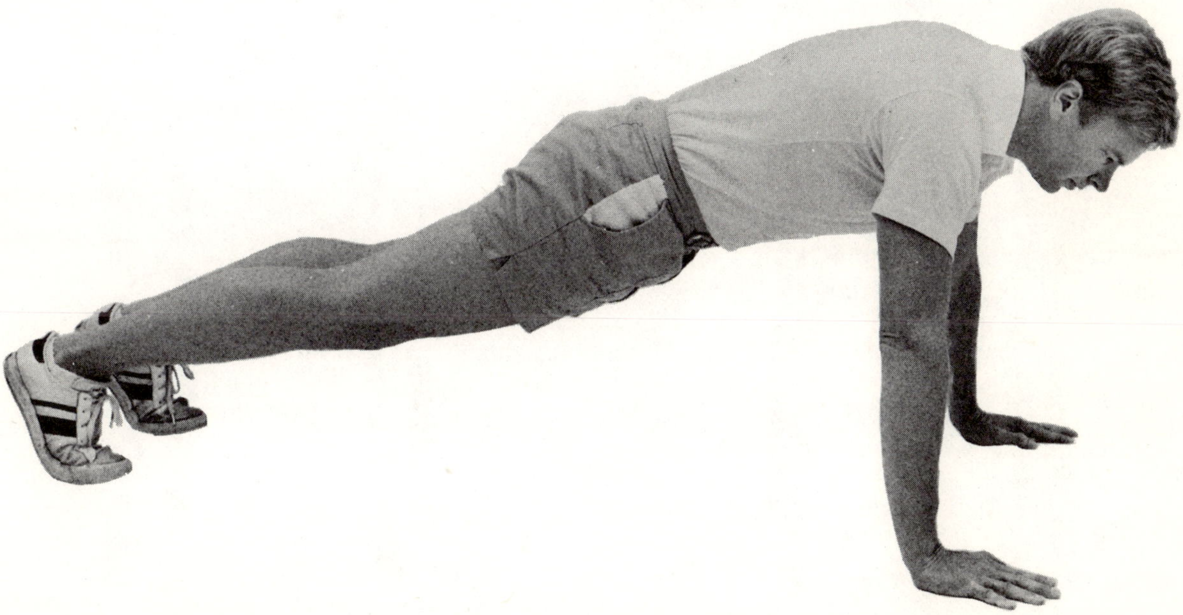

2 Press until arms are straight. Then lower body until you almost touch floor. Go up and down perhaps 5 times, not touching floor until you rest at end of set.

Advanced Push-Up

(Strengthening)

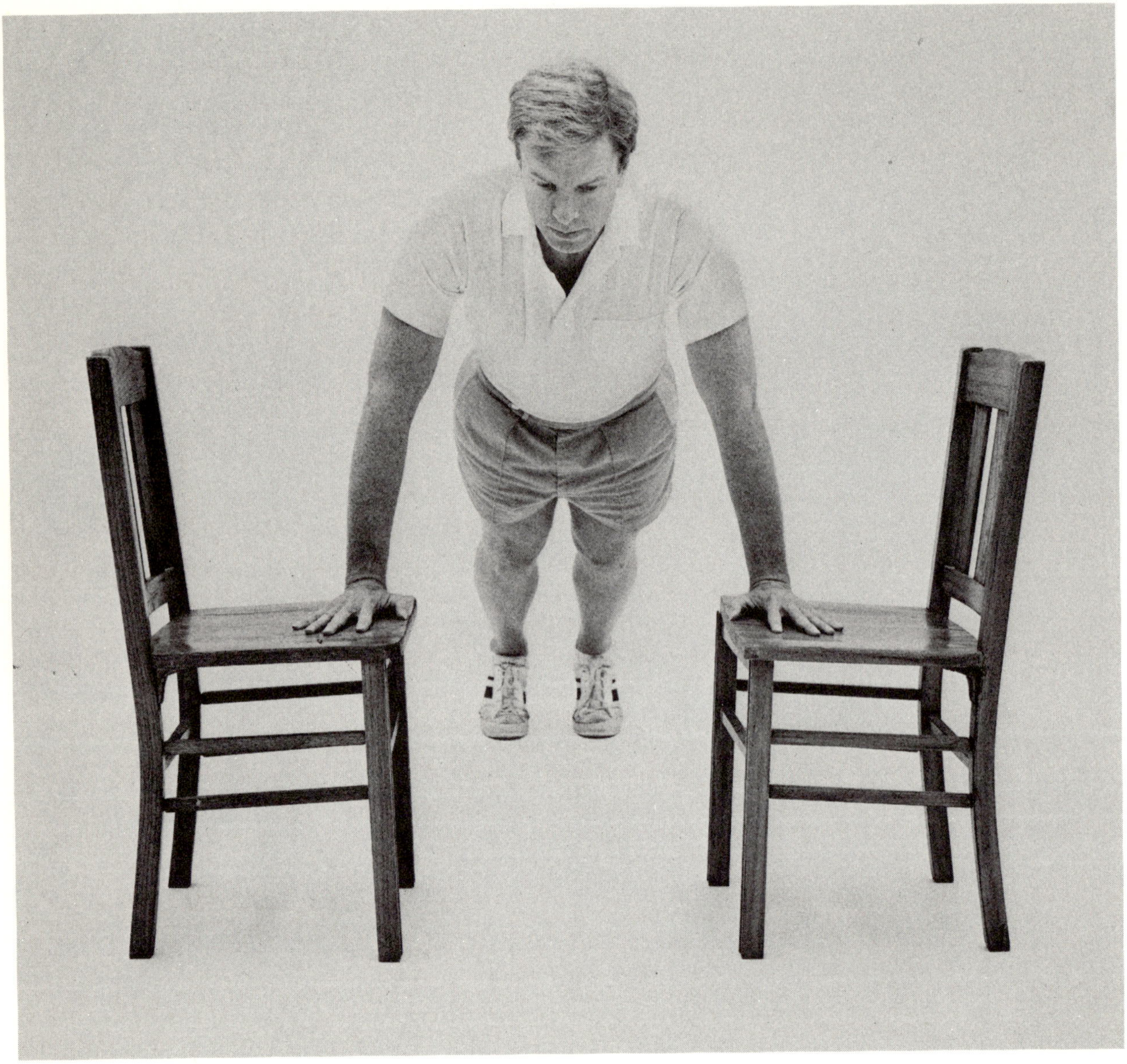

1 **Arms straight, plant hands squarely on chair seats with thumb of either hand beneath edge of shoulder.**

This is *only for the most advanced pupils* and should be done slowly and under full control to avoid excessive stress on the breastbone. Two sturdy chairs are required. Begin as shown, with your entire body and arms straight, hands planted squarely on the chair seats, and the thumb of each hand positioned directly beneath the edge of each shoulder. Now lower your body, keeping it perfectly straight, as far down as you can go. Straighten your arms to return to the original position. Repeat.

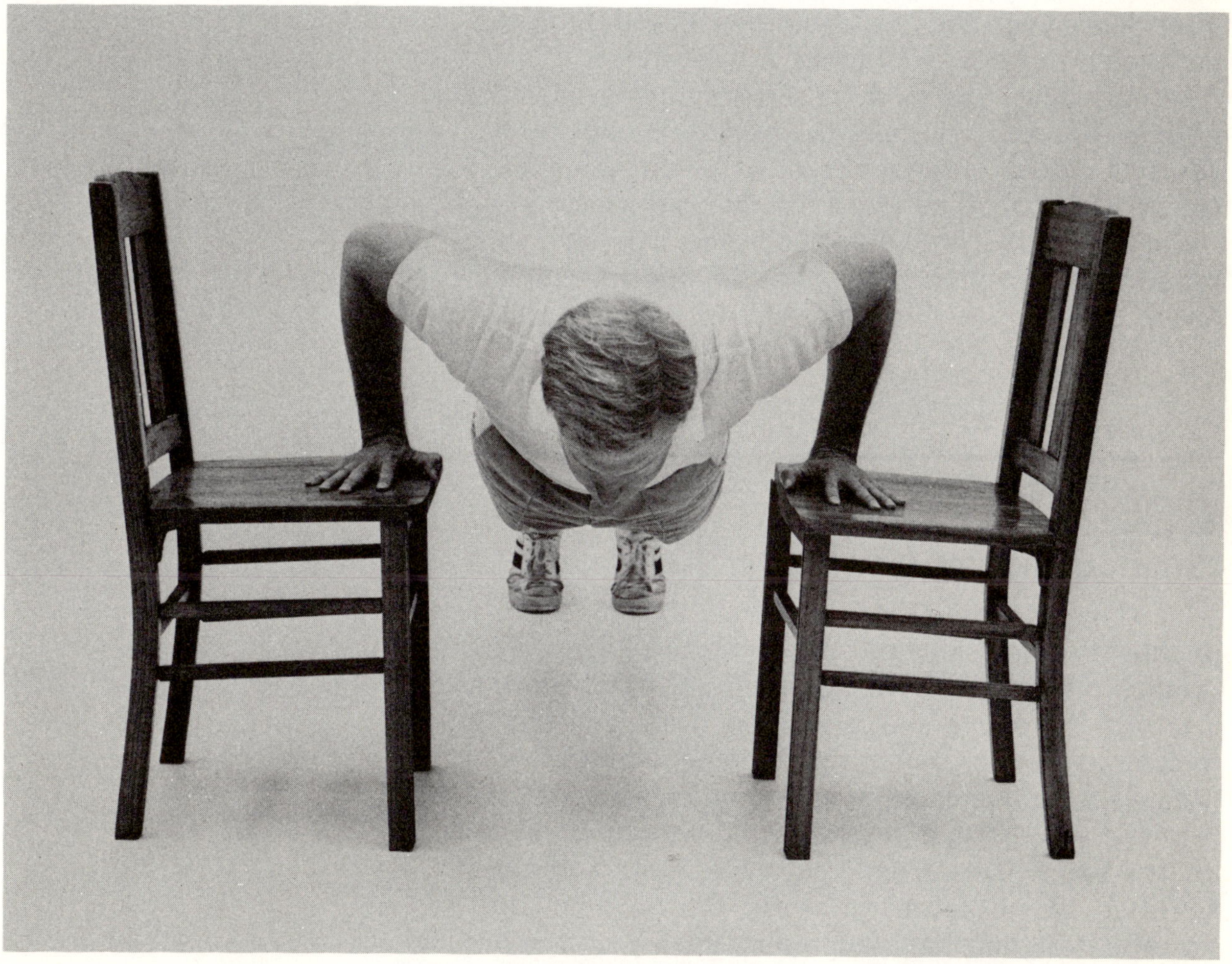

2 Lower body, keeping it straight, as far as you can. Straighten arms to return to original position. Repeat.

Leg Press-Ups

(Strengthening)

This orthopedically sound knee-strengthening exercise requires no expensive, elaborate, specialized equipment—only a few thick books or foot-long sections of board. The object is to exercise your knee by placing your entire weight on the bent leg, then straightening it. You can steady yourself against a wall as needed. First, place one foot on the raised surface. Then bring your body directly over your raised foot and press up, straightening your leg and raising yourself up. Lower the free foot nearly to the floor, but *do not let it touch the floor*. Raise your body up again by straightening the bent leg. Repeat 5 to 10 times with each leg.

Gradually, in successive exercises, increase both the number of repetitions and the height. Do not push yourself. Add additional boards or books, use a footstool, or stand by the stairs. Be sure whatever you stand on is *very stable*. Eventually you will have your raised foot some 15 to 17 inches off the floor (advanced level).

Leg Lift

(Strengthening)

A substitute (not illustrated) for the Leg Press-Up is available for persons with problem knees who can't perform the above exercise. This is the Leg Lift, often recommended for persons with damaged knee cartilage. While sitting in a chair, extend one leg straight out in front of you. Hang a 1- or 2-pound weight (sand in a plastic bag will do) from your ankle. Raise and lower your leg. Do not let it rest on the floor. Do not bother to raise it higher than your waist; keep your leg parallel to the floor at the top of the raise. Begin with 5 or more repetitions, and increase the number and weight as your knee is strengthened.

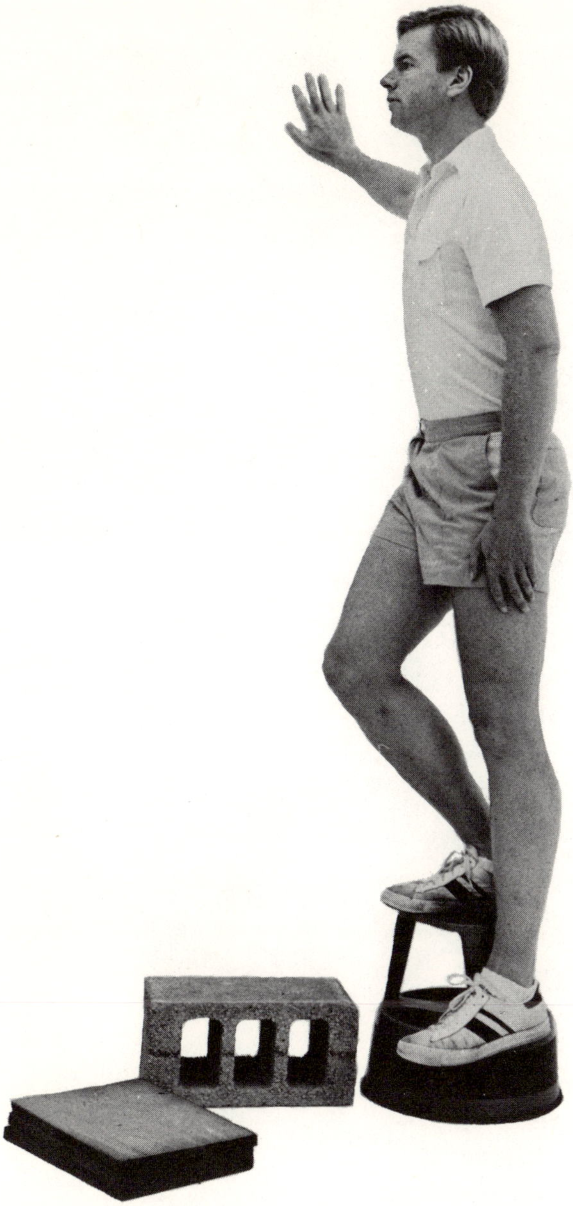

1 Step up onto block or stool (plank: beginner level; block: intermediate; stool: advanced). Then place entire weight on bent leg and slowly straighten it.

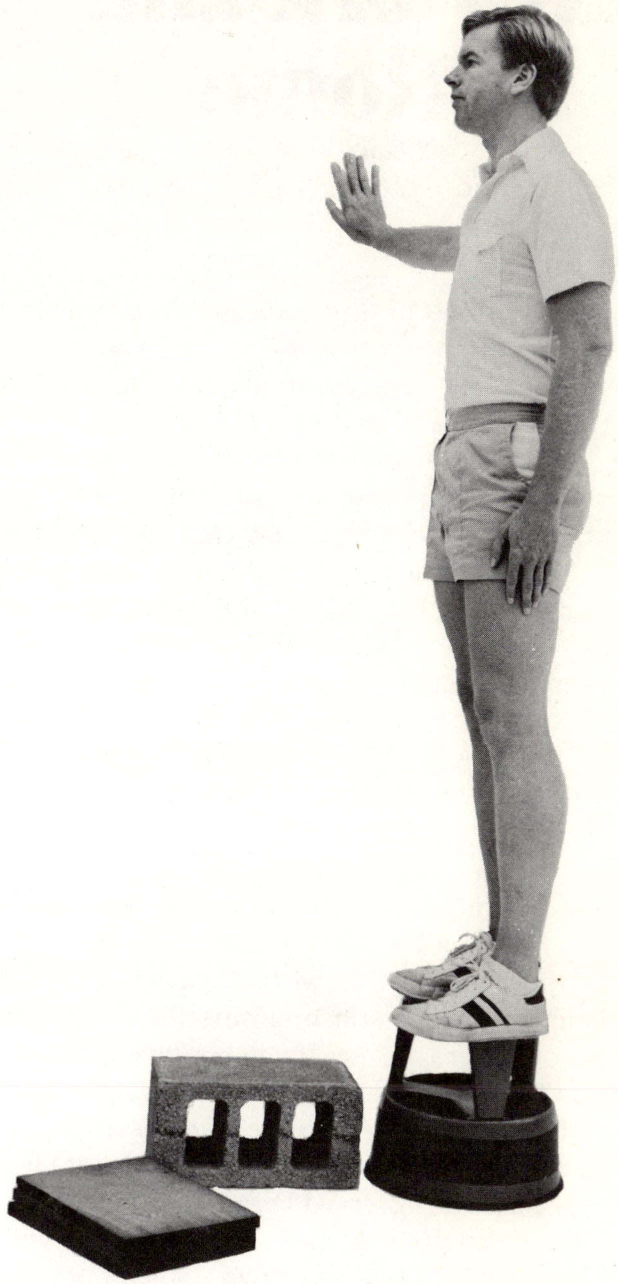

2 When both legs are at same height, lower "off" leg *almost* to floor without touching. Then raise it again. Do this 5 to 10 times for each leg. Gradually you can do more.

At Work and at Home

The exercises in this book involve nearly every bodily action you experience as you function throughout each day at work and at home. The cardinal principle and basic premise of this program is that FITness must relate to daily functions and not to a set of FEATS. The exercises already described serve to reduce your fatigue and increase your stamina and ability to perform everyday tasks without strain or injury.

Let us now consider the daily functions of going to work and working at home. Customarily, there is a frantic, last-minute search for this and that. The briefcase, overcoat, hat, and car keys are gathered up by the harried junior executive going to work or the pressured homemaker on the way to the supermarket. They start the day under tension. The first rule, therefore, is give yourself enough time to get started in the morning to eliminate that frantic, last-minute rush.

Often it is when we abruptly demand the unexpected from our bodies that pain and strain result. Bending, lifting, and twisting with a heavy suitcase or even a briefcase may result in a muscle spasm, a spinal disk problem, or the like. If you condition yourself to "reach down with your legs" by bending at the knees, you will minimize, if not eliminate, the possibility of hurting your back. In fact, every opportunity for reaching down with your legs must be observed throughout every day.

As you are driving to the office, you will undoubtedly encounter a red light or two. Instead of fuming about the delay, use the time to do a good abdominal exercise. Exhale and seek to draw your stomach back to your spine. The abdominal area of most people is notoriously flabby and soft. Observing this simple procedure while driving can do wonders for the muscle tone of the abdominal wall. The PE coach used to scream at you, "Suck in that gut!" Well, all these years later, you're now doing it and voluntarily at that! Push back hard just with your abdominal muscles, and

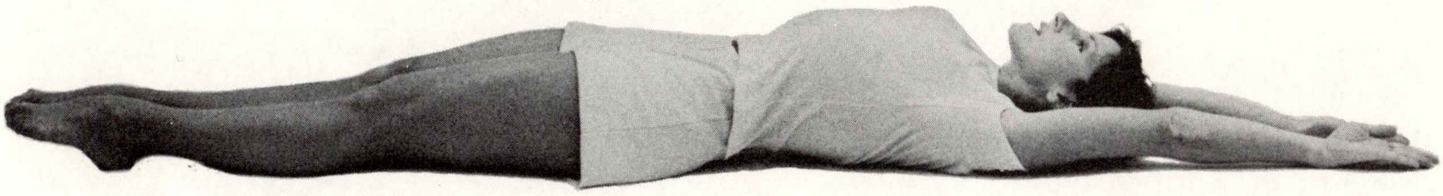

relax your arms and legs. By the time you've done this, the light will probably have changed and you'll be on your way.

At the Office

Assuming that your work at the office is largely sedentary, the tension that you experience will be largely psychological in nature. This is not to imply that it is not *real* tension, simply because it is psychological. It is often assumed that psychological tension is not true tension; it is just a state of mind. Nonsense. Psychological tension can and often does have pronounced physical effects that must be coped with effectively.

In response to this reality, the typical solution in the business community is what is known as the "coffee break," an opportunity for conversation and relaxation. An alternative—or supplement—is an "exercise break" that can give your system the true relaxation that it craves. Tension has been building; it is time for a creative release.

If doing exercises in an office environment would make you feel conspicuous, and you don't have a private office, solve the problem by inviting a coworker or two to join you in these routines. That will make it more acceptable, and you may start a trend! Group exercise in office settings is gaining in popularity.

Typist's Neck Pull

(Strengthening and Loosening)

If you work in an office, you may have to do a lot of typing. Typists frequently complain of painful neck and back-of-the-head aches. Homemakers who have to do a lot of ironing often have the same experience. The Neck Pull, which was shown previously as part of the daily exercises, not only strengthens but relaxes the neck muscles, where tension headaches originate.

While seated, back straight, interlock fingers and hands high on the back of your head. Slowly and steadily pull forward with your arms, but at the same time stiffen the neck so as to defeat the forward pull. Maintain tension for 30 seconds or so, then relax by removing your hands, dropping them to your side, and allowing your head to drop down. Try to touch your chin to your body. Resume normal head position and repeat the exercise 2 or 3 times.

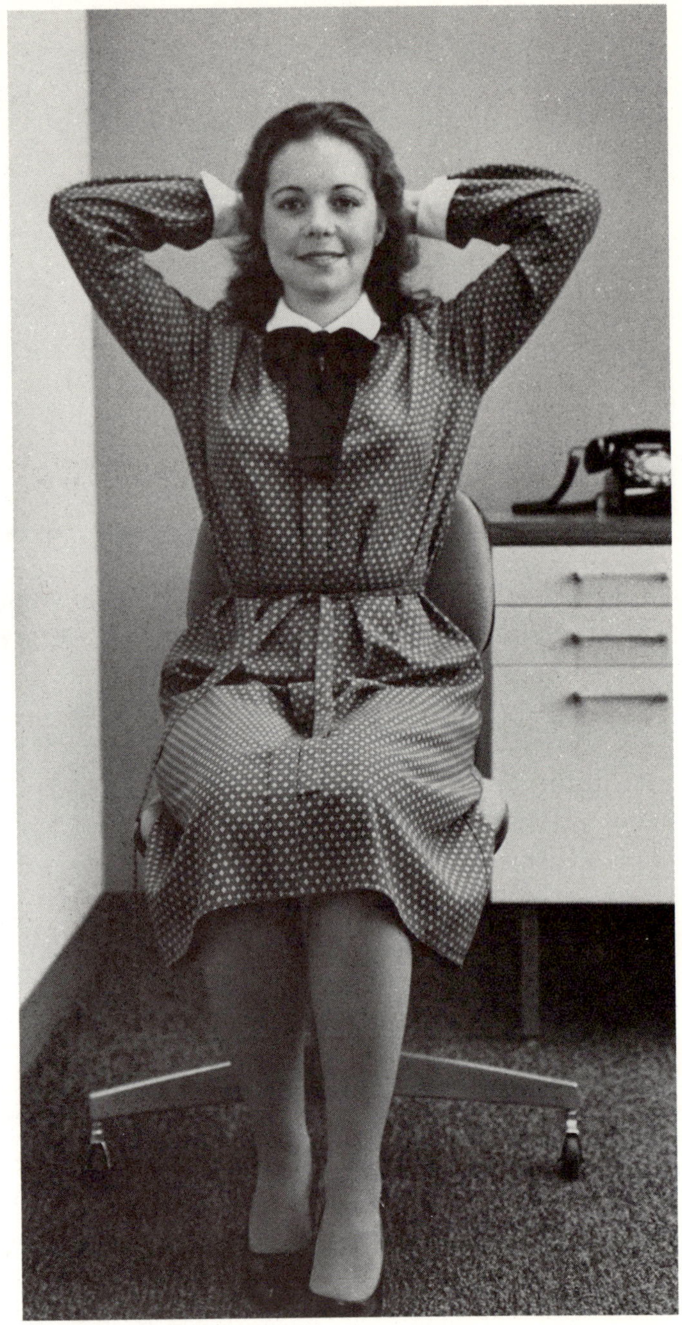

1 Sit erect in chair with hands interlocked on back of head.

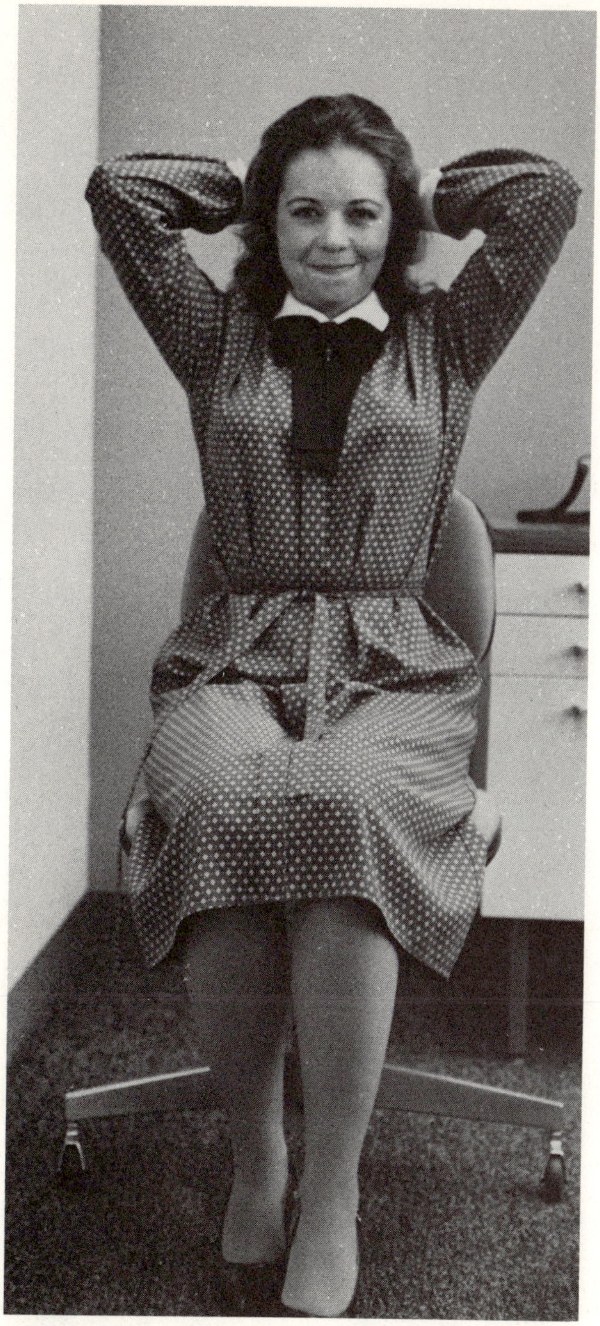

2 Pull forward with arms but stiffen neck and push back with head to resist forward pull. Hold 30 seconds, then relax.

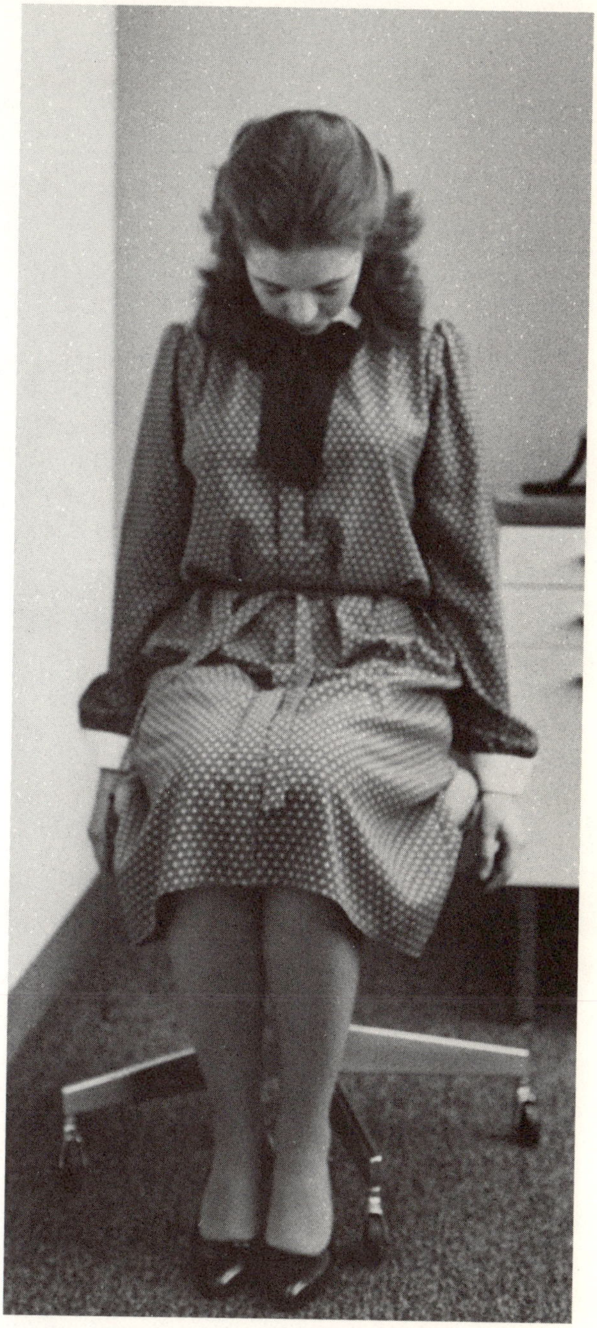

3 Remove hands, drop them to your side and drop chin to chest. Relax. Repeat this exercise 2 to 3 times.

Typist's Shrug

(Loosening)

The Shrug is a good exercise for one who must type a great amount each day. While sitting in your chair, let your hands and arms fall to your sides, then roll your shoulders up and around. In short, shrug your shoulders. This gives needed change and relief to those long muscles that run from the neck to the shoulders, the trapezius muscles. The added circulation and motion tend to bring relief after hours of typing. Try it; it does help.

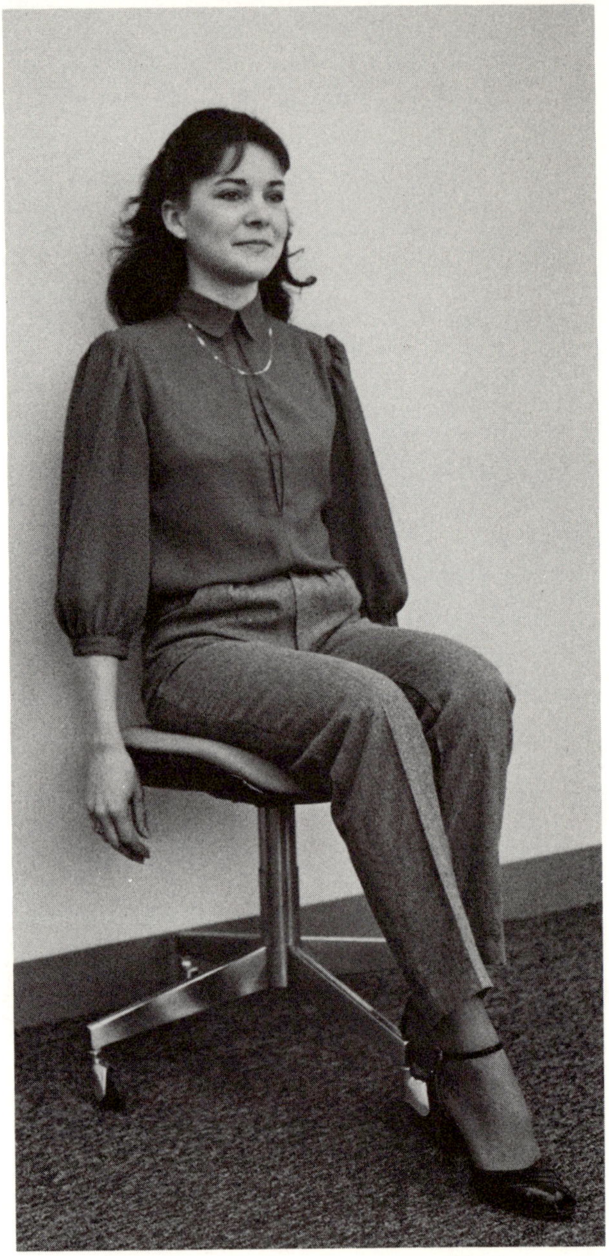

1 Sit erect in armless chair, arms hanging down loosely.

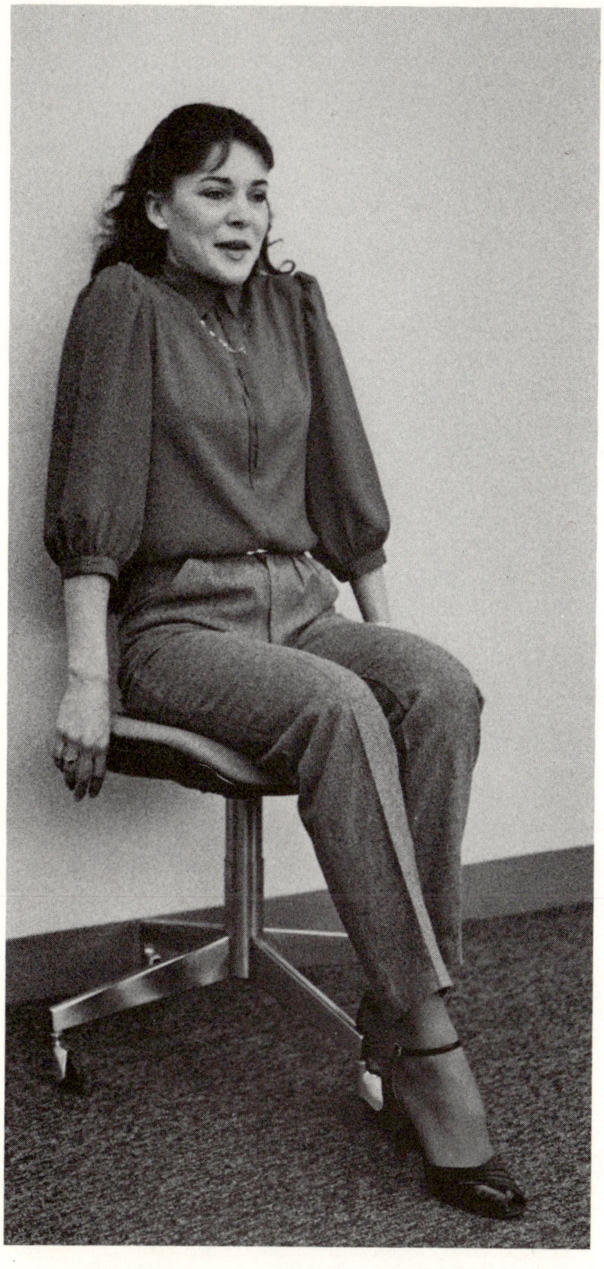

2 Slowly roll your shoulders up and forward.

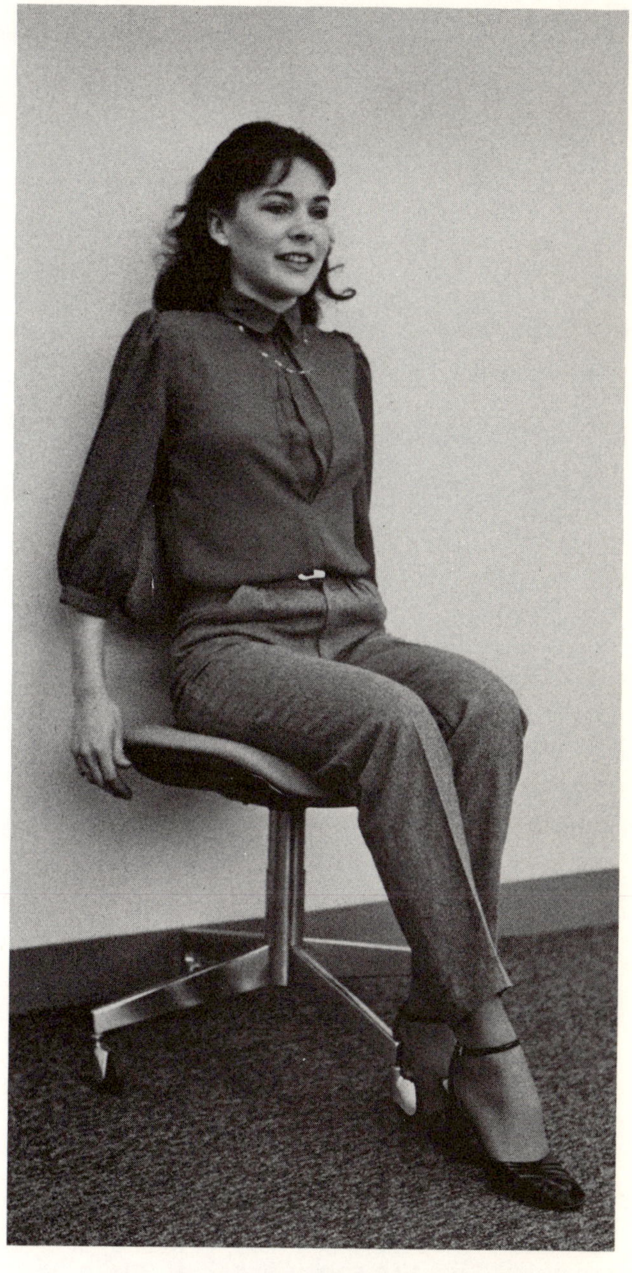

3 Roll your shoulders back and into original position. Repeat exercise 2 to 3 times.

Coffee-Break Relaxer

(Stretching/Firming)

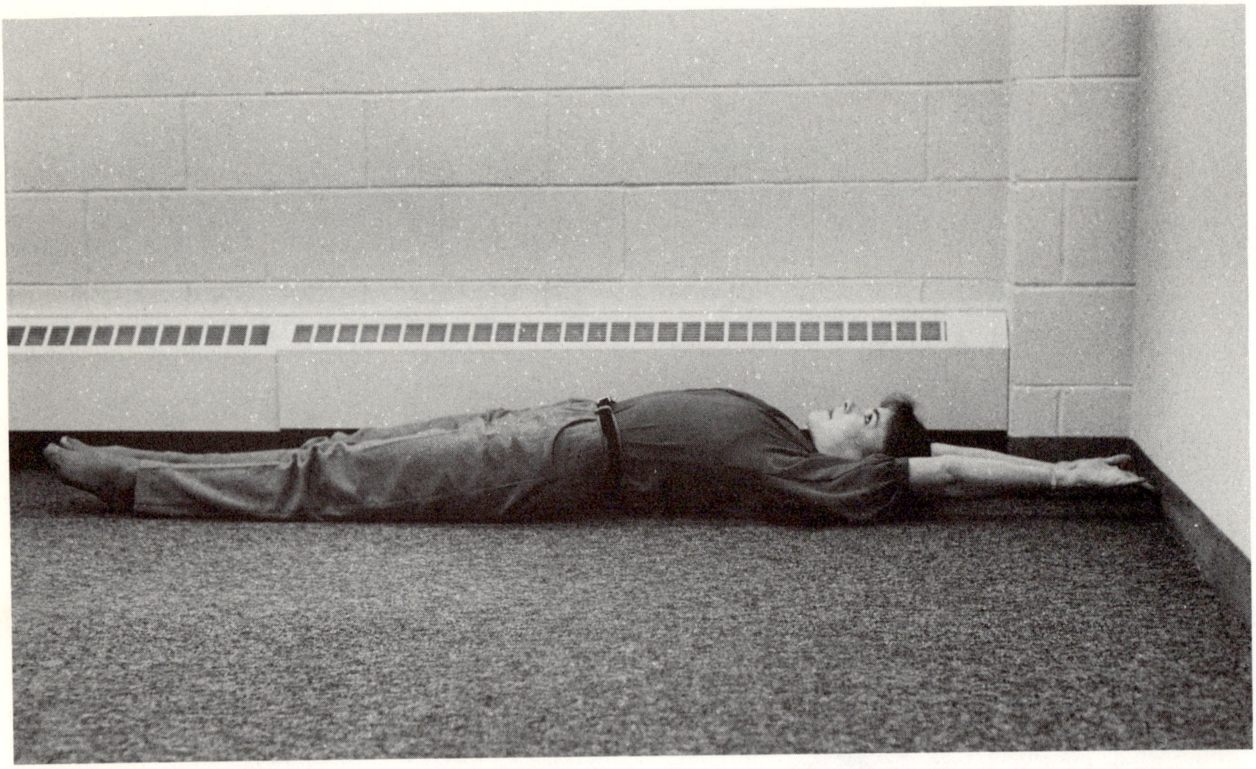

1 Lying on back, try to reach wall behind you while pointing toes and stretching legs. Exhale and try to draw your stomach back to your spine.

Another good coffee-break exercise for tension release is available to those who have access to a private space. Simply lie on your back and extend your arms backward and stretch and stretch and stretch. Remember the abdominal exercise you did in the car? After a few stretches, do the same exercise while lying on your back. Exhale and seek to draw your stomach back to your spine. You can conclude the exercise by drawing both knees up to your chest.

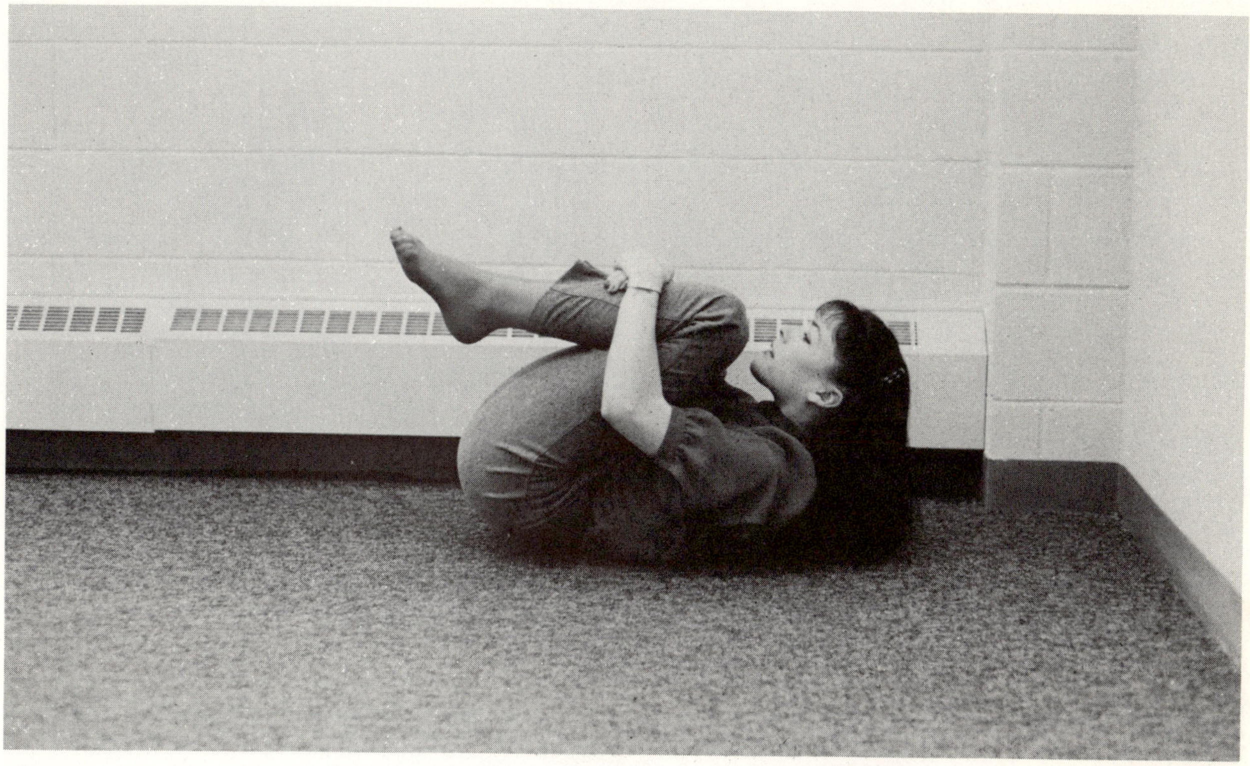

2 Conclude exercise by wrapping arms around knees, knees to chin, and curling up in a ball.

Saving Your Back at the Office

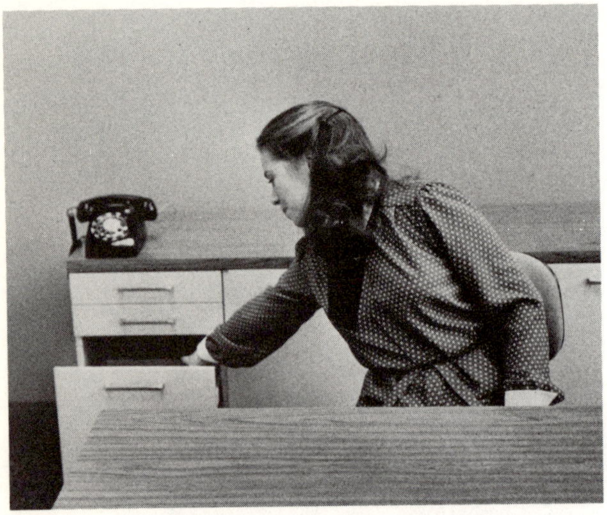

Twisting like this to reach a file can wrench the back.

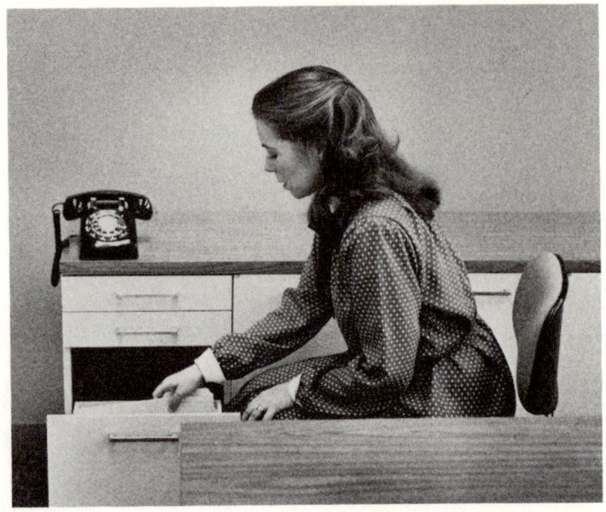

A turn of the chair lets you reach without twisting or bending back.

In most jobs, you do not have to do any lifting of consequence during the normal day. If you should, and even though it may be nothing more than a few chairs in the conference room, observe the fundamentals of lifting with your legs rather than with your back. Position yourself and make ready to lift rather than just rushing to get the chair moved. Similarly, when you bend down to open a file drawer, *bend at the knees*. And, when you reach for something, be careful not to twist your body. These are simple reminders, but when overlooked, a debilitating muscle spasm can result.

Think before you lift. Plan before you lift. Always start by asking yourself this question: "How can I lift this without bending my back?" Once you have established your grasp and before you begin your lift, bring your head to the upright position. Look ahead, raise your body up (beginning with your legs), and keep your back straight.

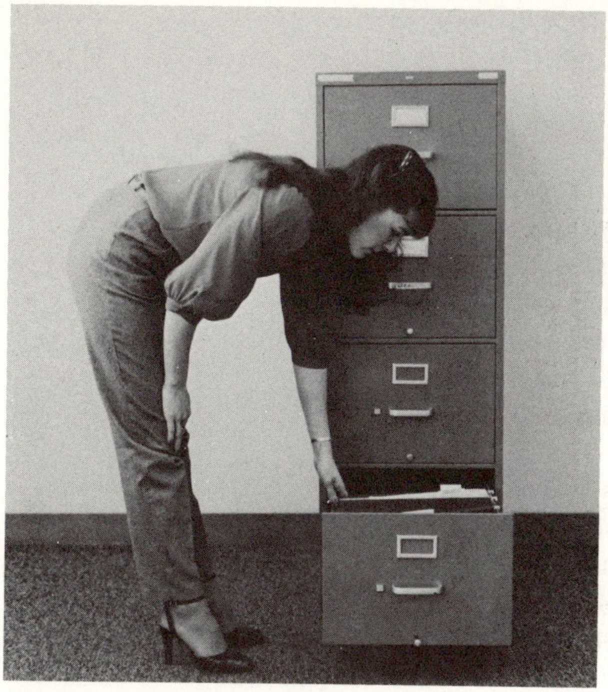

Bending over like this to reach down is the wrong approach. It puts a strain on lower back.

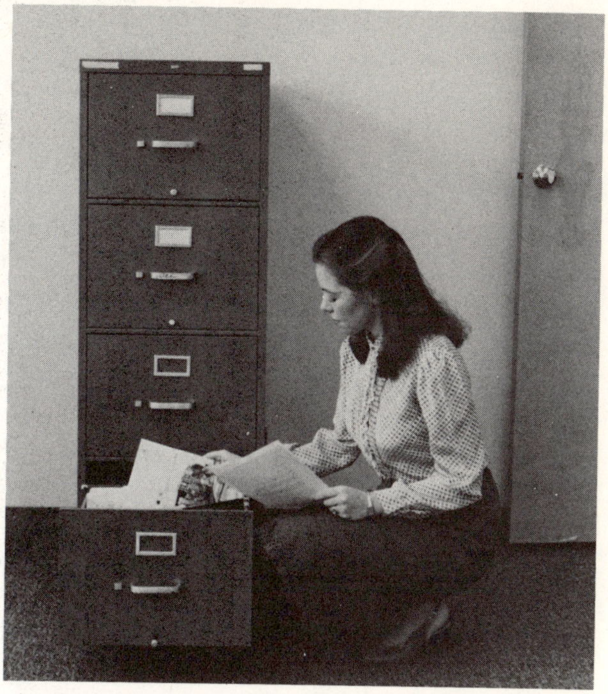

Bend with the legs, not the back when you have to get something out of a lower file drawer.

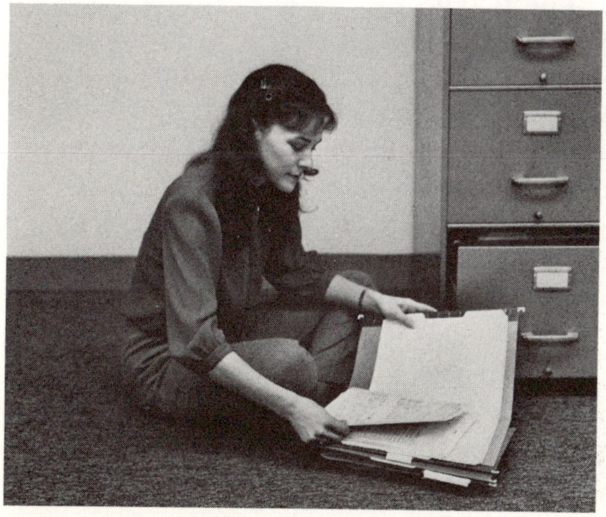

If the bent-legs posture becomes tiring, sit on the floor to examine material from files.

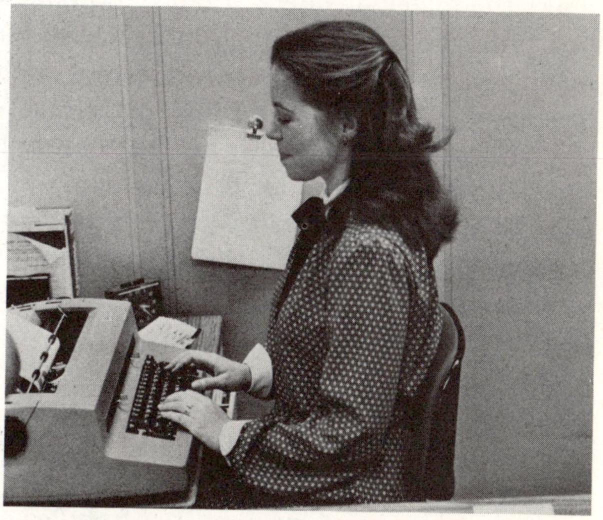

Good posture while typing helps to prevent aches of the back, shoulder, and neck.

At Home

Now for the person whose workload is mainly at home. Everything from lifting the laundry basket to sweeping the floor or making a bed can be either a hazard or good exercise, depending on how you do it. If you bear in mind that you are going to attempt to keep your back reasonably straight throughout the performance of all household tasks, you have made the right start.

One of the basic problems in housework is the tendency to view all of the duties of the home as those belonging to "the little woman." The women's rights movement has done much to expose this fallacy and the injustice of it. Many women, however, have continued to shoulder much of the heavy work in the home, when they should enlist the aid of another person for heavy lifting or moving.

There are a number of simple things that you can do to make your work easier while protecting your back at the same time. Assuming that you have a broom and a mop as two of the heavy weapons in your arsenal of home-aids, make the following check: Hold the broom with the tip just touching the floor. The top of the broom handle should reach your chin, but I'll bet it does not. Now, I'm not going to suggest that you buy a handle stretcher or anything like that. Simply lengthen your present broom handle by taking the handle of a discarded broom, mop, or waxing mop, and tape it firmly to your good broom handle at such a point as to make it long enough to reach your chin. You will be amazed that you can sweep easier and better without even bending over at all!

When it comes time to pick up the debris, bend the legs as opposed to bending at the waist (or use a dustpan with a long handle). What is good for the broom is also good for the mop and the rake.

It is indeed unfortunate that handles on brooms, mops, and rakes are so short. You will find it much easier to mop if you use a longer handle. As with raking and sweeping, a good rule to follow with mopping is to stay close to the area

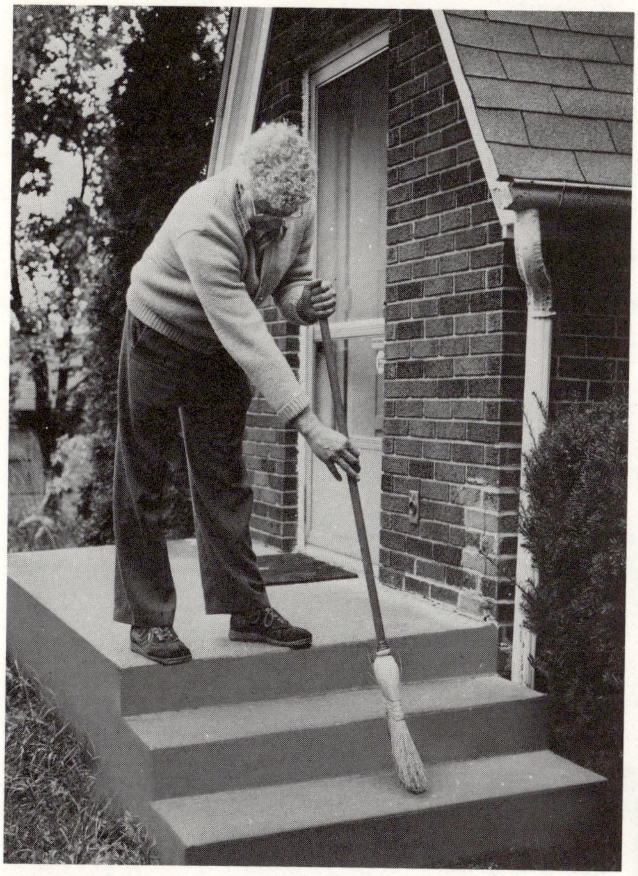

Bending over to sweep stairs could hurt your back.

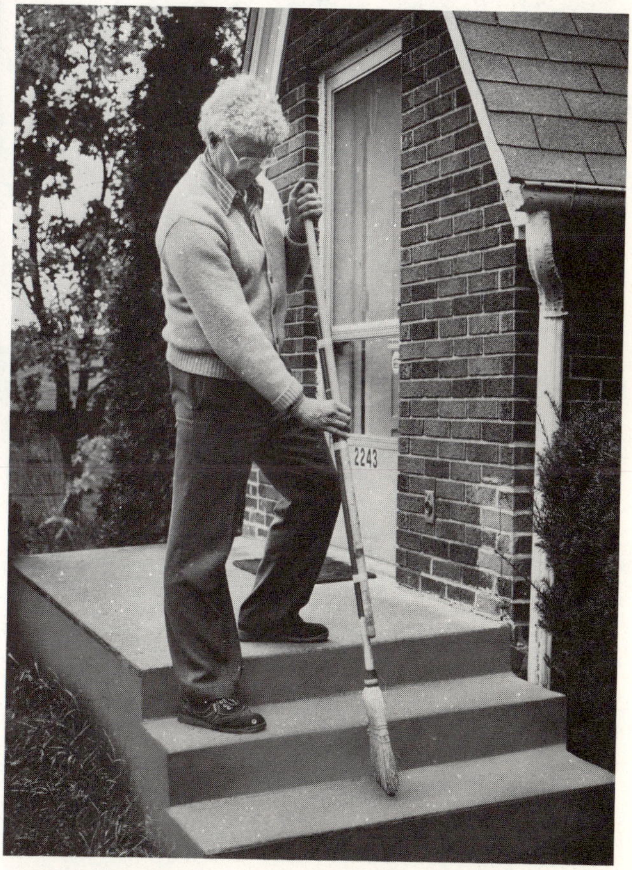

Broom-handle extension lets you sweep without bending.

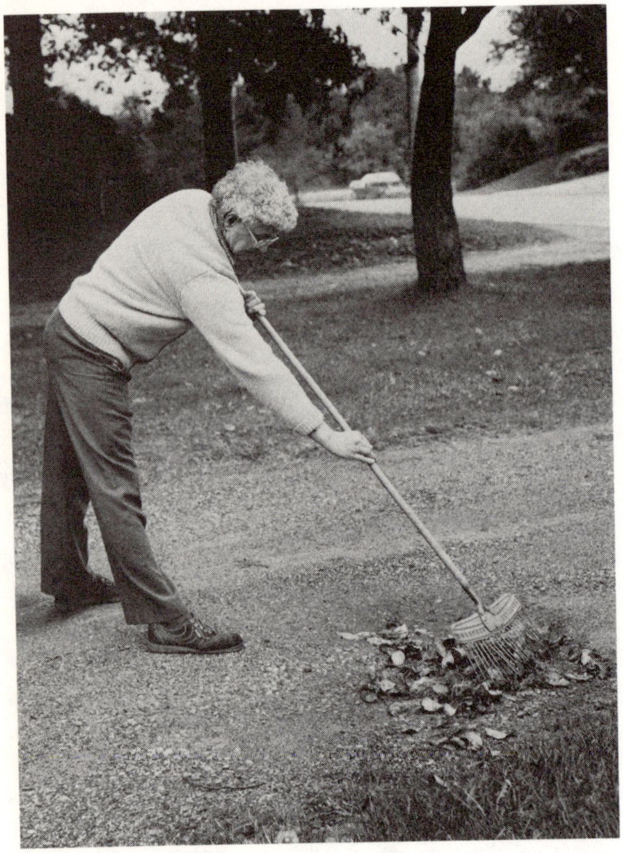

Reach like this when you're raking and you could hurt your back by excessive bending.

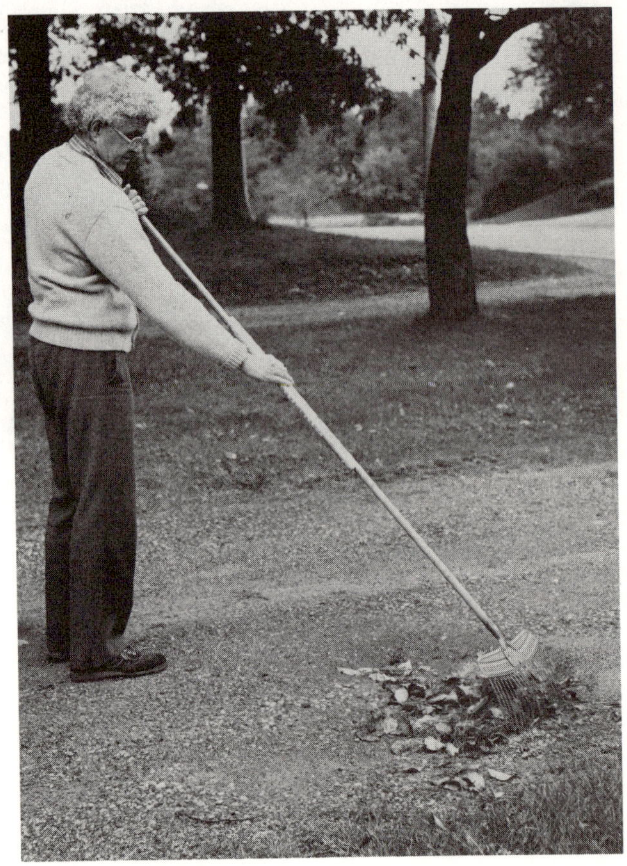

Lengthen the rake handle and you can reach just as far without bending the back.

being mopped rather than stretching halfway across the room to reach the area not yet done. Always mop side to side, left to right, right to left, while moving backwards away from the area mopped. This way you will be able to stand reasonably straight throughout the entire operation.

For some reason, people who vacuum seem to behave as if their feet were nailed to the floor! Move to the area to be vacuumed, and maintain an erect posture while vacuuming. When you vacuum the stairs, start at the top. If you're using an upright vacuum, lock it in the upright position, stand on the step below, and proceed *down* one step at a time. Do not try to vacuum up the stairs, reaching farther and farther until something snaps or seizes in your back.

The automatic washer and dryer have revolutionized the home laundry operation. I have often observed persons at the laundromat, however, testing their backs by failing either to sit by the dryer to unload it or not bending the knees while removing the load. If the washer or dryer is front-loading, it is easy to forget to sit or bend the knees to unload it. This can result in back strain and even injury. Lifting a heavy basket of wet laundry requires the same precaution as lifting any other heavy load. It can be made easier if the basket is on a chair or stool when it is being filled. In this way, you do not have to reach down to the floor to lift up the basket. This is a very simple adjustment, but it will lighten the load on your back considerably.

Stooping over is a bad habit and should be avoided at all times. Sit and fold the laundry. Wouldn't it be nice if the front-loading machines were at the same height as the counter in your kitchen? It's not a bad idea, but don't look for it to happen overnight. It will be necessary for you to adjust to the height of the machine and not vice versa.

Those of you with top-loading machines must be wondering what you can do. It seems almost impossible to reach down into a machine without having to bend at the waist with the legs straight. It is difficult, but the basic rule is to remember to reach in several times and not try to remove all of the wet clothes at one time in one big lift. Also, if you stand sideways to the machine and bend your knees, you can reach inside the washer very easily without having to bend at the waist. People sometimes complain that they cannot see what they're doing if this posture is adopted. Well, what it is that they must look for? The clothes they put in the machine are still there, and they will be located quickly enough.

When it is time to take the laundry upstairs, let's hope you have not made a closet of your stairs! People who put things on stairs, saving them for later trips, often forget and find the items with their feet in the dark or when their vision is blocked by a laundry basket. Avoid using stairs as shelves or closets. Either take the item up or down or leave it someplace else. All of those cartoon jokes about falls on roller skates or other items left on stairs are not in the least bit funny in real life!

It is true that because of the new permanent-press fabrics, ironing is virtually a lost art for many people. If you still do some ironing, however, remember this: *Don't stand up when you're ironing*. Sit down! Bending over an ironing board can give you an aching back, and it's unnecessary. Most ironing boards today can be adjusted in height to permit you to sit while ironing. It's far more comfortable. You don't bend your back. There's no disadvantage in motion, because you simply slide the ironing board around a bit as you iron instead of moving about the work area. Try it. You will be pleasantly surprised at how much easier the task becomes.

Bringing home the groceries is a thankless, taxing, and difficult job which is often made worse by the trunk design of many cars. When the floor of the vehicle's storage area is level with the opening, as in a station wagon, the task is greatly simplified. If, however, you have a traditional trunk, your grocery bags are nestled deep in the well of the trunk, and your work is greatly increased. You must bend over and down to grasp the bags. You will lift them from the bottom because of what happened when you tried top-lifting and the bottom fell out of the bag!

It appears that by virtue of the trunk's design you are

going to have to bend your back, and your profile will become the hairpin you have been trying to avoid! This is not necessary at all. Keep a few large canvas beach bags or strong plastic shopping bags in the trunk. Put the bags of groceries in these containers which have handles on the top so that you don't have to bend over much in order to lift them out.

When you consider the amount of time spent bringing home groceries in the course of a year, it is indeed wise to make such provisions to ease the load. Obviously, a station wagon body style is the easiest to load and a deep trunk the worst. Adjust to your vehicle as suggested. You should never let the trunk dictate to your back!

A household task that often sends a person to the orthopedist is moving and rearranging the furniture. Most people do this on impulse and without careful preplanning. It's often discovered that something "doesn't fit here after all," and hence the lifting and shifting goes on and on.

Always begin your moving with a tape measure. It helps settle arguments without moving the article in question to the desired spot to see whether it fits or not. Obvious as this may seem, many people overlook it, and the result is a harassed couple wandering around the room with a sofa between them, trying it here, there, and everywhere. Know in advance where you want to go with a piece of furniture, and make sure it will fit there before you lift it. In the actual lifting, be sure to bend with the legs, keeping the back straight. Plan your move out in advance, and then move slowly, yet surely. Lift together, take your time, and be sure you're loosened up and ready to lift. This is quite important.

You see athletes loosen up before a race, match, or game, and with good reason. Being "cold" does not mean that you necessarily *feel cold*; it means that your muscles are not prepared for the extra demands you are about to make of them. Stretch a bit, flex, and be sure your shoes are stable and give good support. If you are concerned as to whether you are "cold" or not, take a minute and do the Dancer's exercise and the Knee-to-Chest exercise before engaging in the lifting.

Bringing Home the Groceries

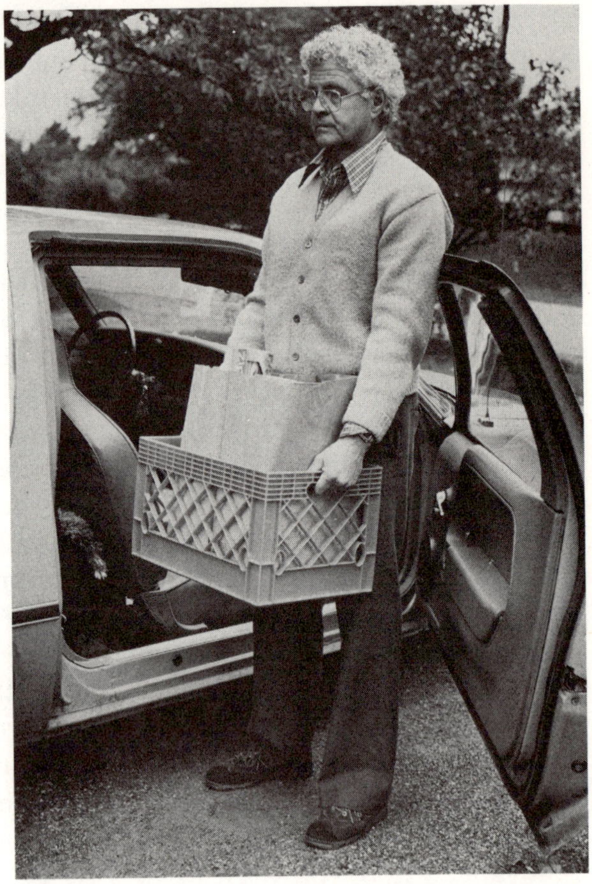

Place your bags of groceries in a box with handholds.

One way to prevent the wrenched back that may result from lifting groceries out of a deep car trunk is to *not use the trunk* for this purpose but to place the groceries in a box on the passenger seat beside you. The box could be a lightweight plastic crate (as shown) that you can buy, or it could be a homemade box that provides a little loop or slot which will accommodate the passenger seat belt. This will hold the groceries secure, in the event that you must stop suddenly.

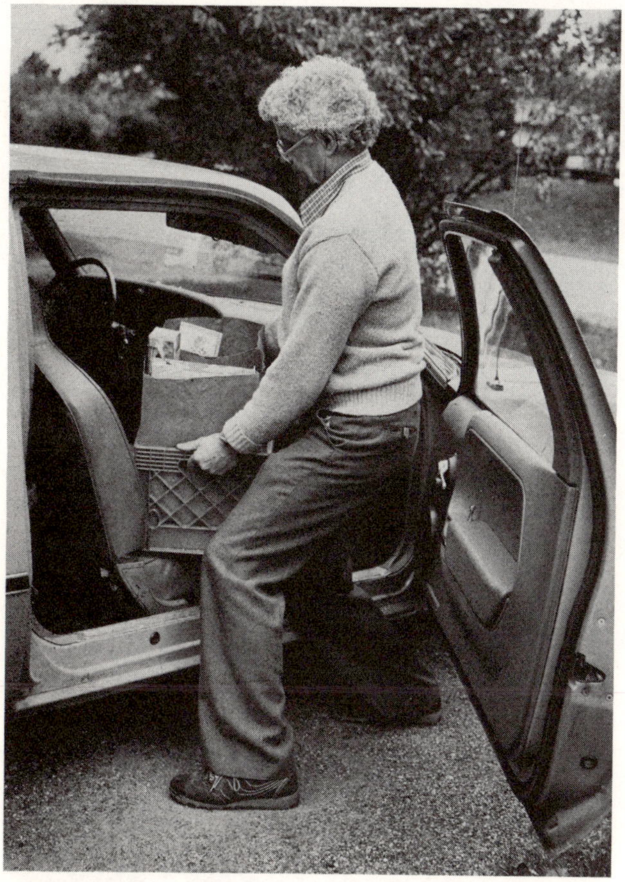

Notice that the back is straight as the box is placed on the front seat of the car beside driver.

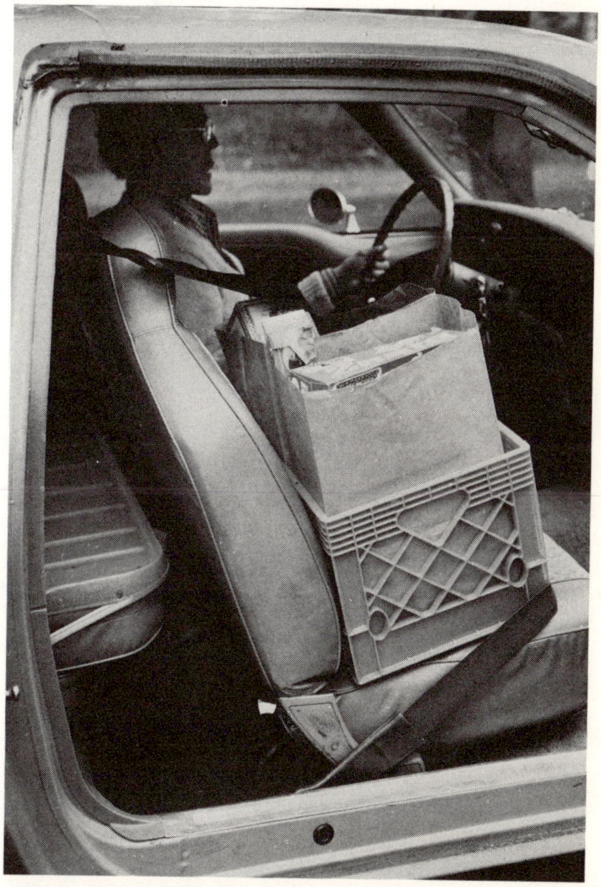

Seat belt holds the grocery box in position. This is a better place to carry groceries than a deep auto trunk.

Right and Wrong Ways to Lift

The importance of protecting your back while lifting cannot be overemphasized. Bend with your legs, not your back. A good rule to follow is to always look straight ahead when lifting. If you look straight in front of you, this keeps your head up. With your head up, you are less likely to bend over. You may need to look down first to see what you are doing. Once you have established your grasp and before you begin to lift, bring your head to the upright position, look ahead, and then raise your body up, beginning with your legs and keeping your back straight.

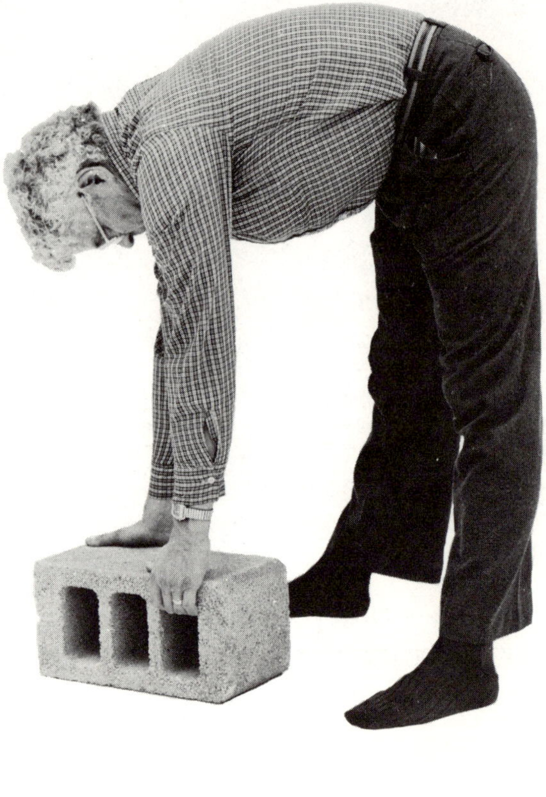

Even with shoes on, this is the wrong way to lift. It puts pressure on the vulnerable lower back.

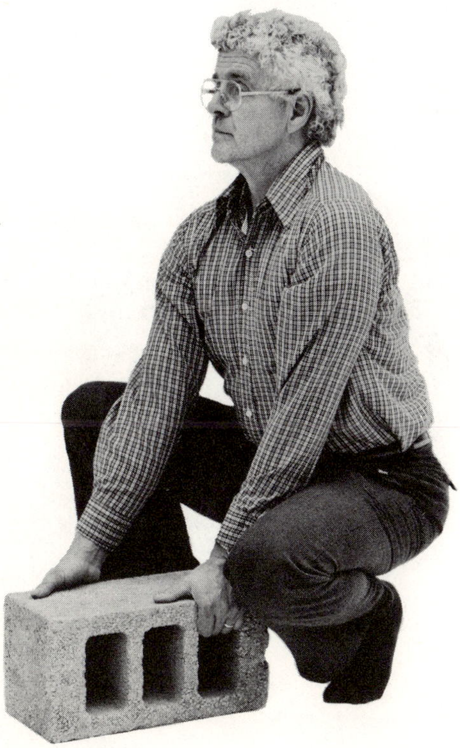

Get as close as possible to the object, bend knees, then look ahead and straighten back as you lift.

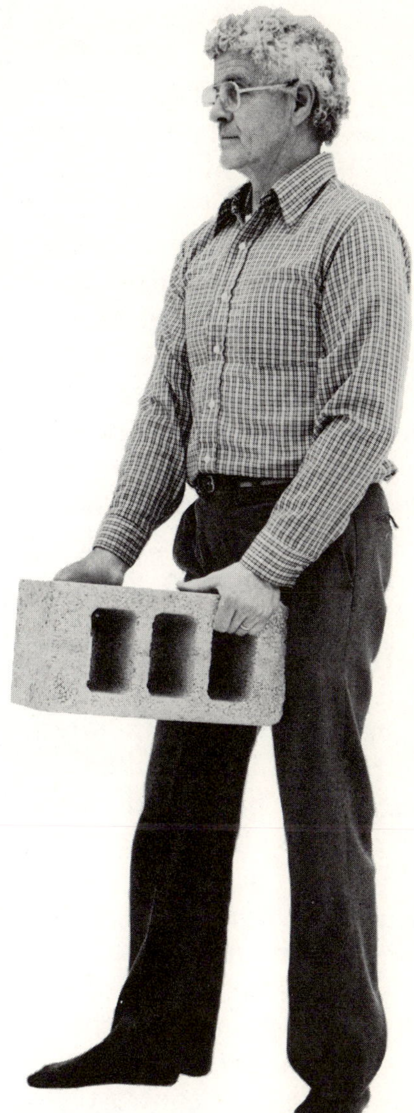

When you lift correctly, with eyes ahead and back straight, your arms and legs do the work, not your back.

Tension Release

(Stretching)

For this good at-home exercise sit in an unupholstered chair. As you count slowly from 1 to 5, extend your arms and legs straight out in front of you. Tense every muscle in your body over which you have voluntary control. When you reach 5, hold it for a second and then start counting back to 1. As you count backwards, slowly but surely lower your arms and legs, releasing the muscles you have tightened until you have eliminated all of the tension in them. When you finish counting backwards, say "zero" and seek to visualize and experience yourself as a total zero, without content or tension whatsoever. Repeat this several times, and you will be delighted to find that it *is* refreshing. Give the exercise your undivided attention. Really concentrate. The contrast between great muscular tension and total relaxation heightens the effect of the relaxation. You may have some trouble achieving full concentration at first, but with practice you will become oblivious to anything but the exercise.

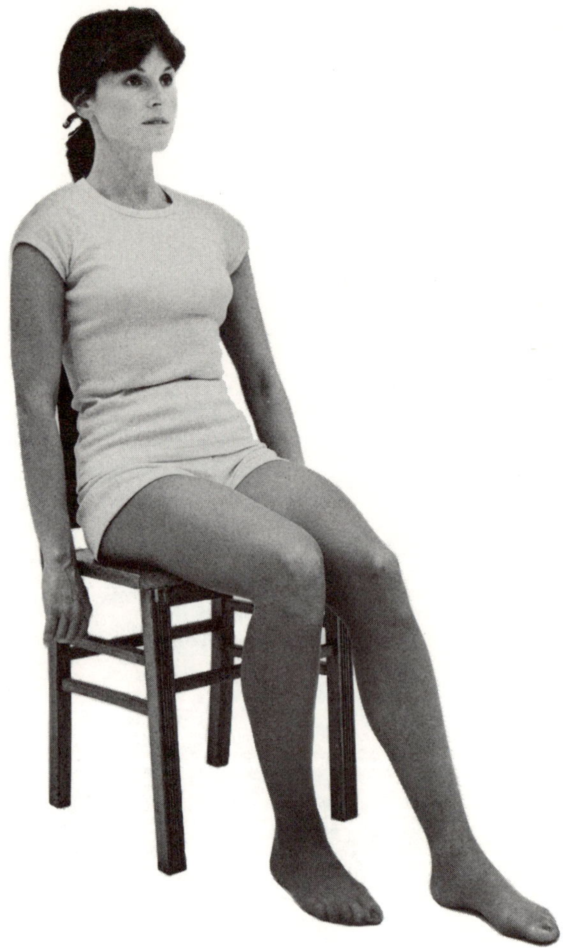

1 Sit erect in straight-back chair, arms hanging at sides.

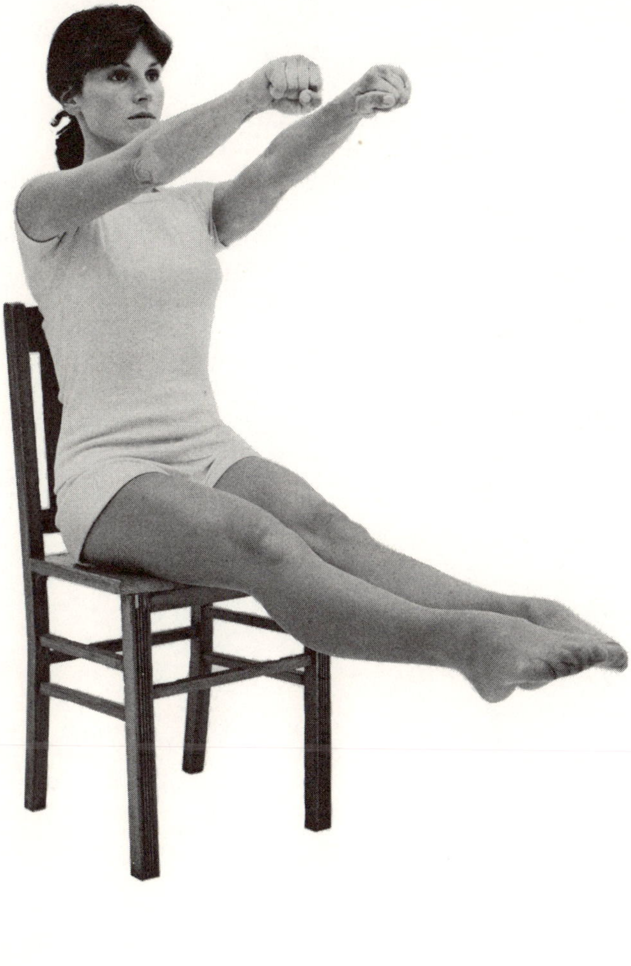

2 Slowly raise arms and legs, making them straighter and stiffer as you count from 1 to 5 (rigid at 5). Pause, then count back to 1, and slowly lower limbs to former positions.

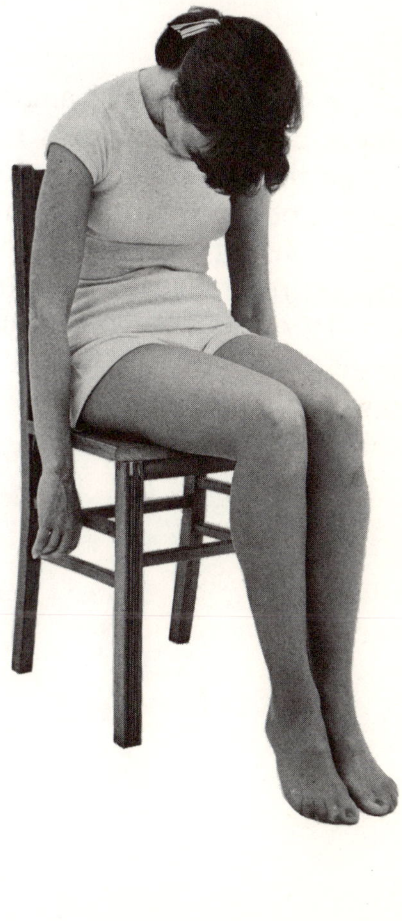

3 Let head and arms fall limp. Release all tension. Learn to turn yourself into Jell-O!

Back Rest

The position shown provides amazing relief for an aching back. It's commonly prescribed for those who have injured their backs and is often the only position in which pain is not felt. But it's also good relaxation for anyone who has a tired back at the end of the day, and it's a way to prevent a backache from developing. You can watch TV or read the newspaper at the same time, while gathering energy for dinner preparation or an evening out.

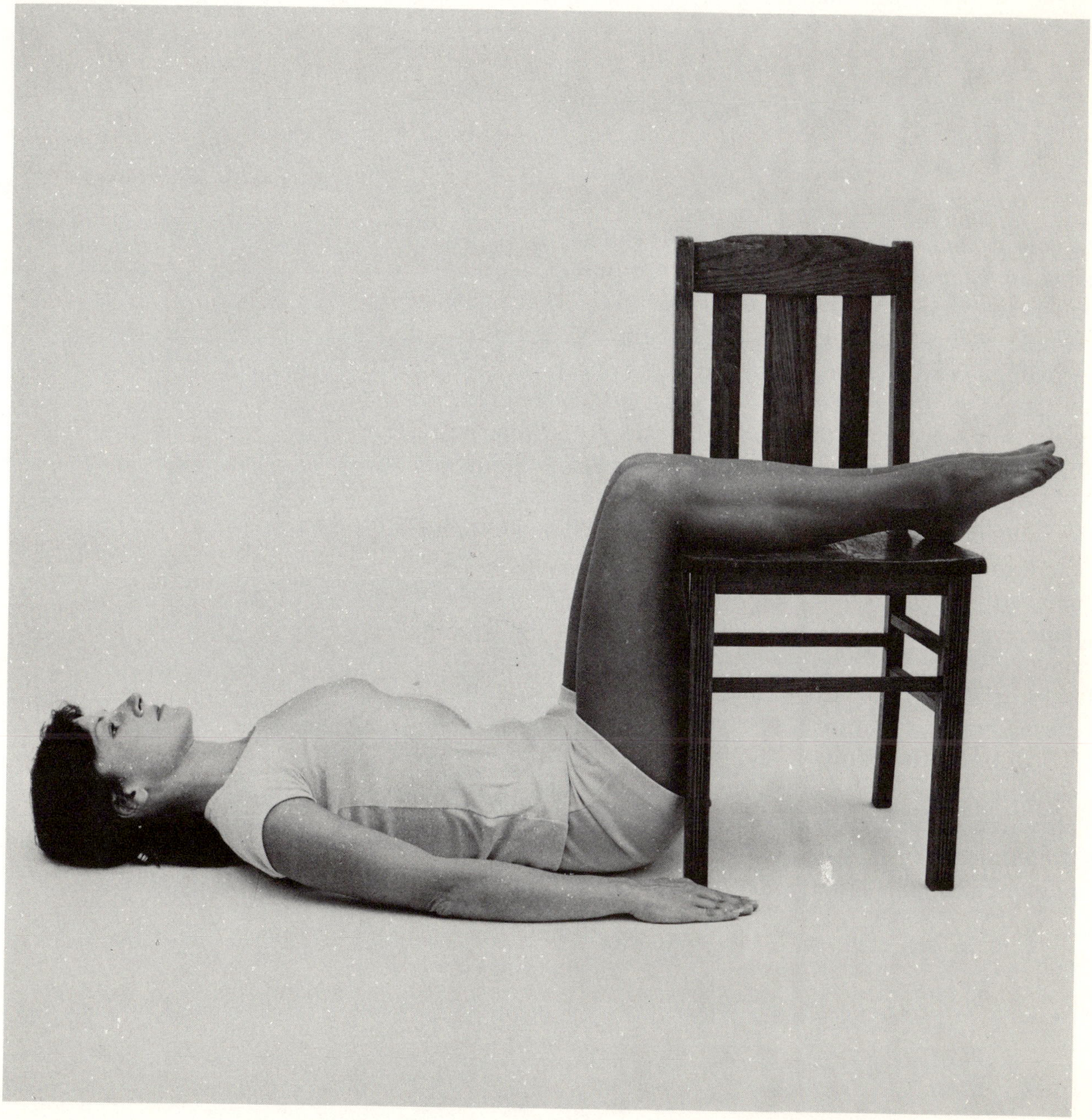

For a relaxing treat, good for an aching back, lie flat on back, legs at right angles resting on chair or sofa.

Body Building with Rubber Bands

An Option

If you are one of those individuals who does best with specific exercises involving simple equipment, let me introduce you to the rubber-band program. Incredibly simple, virtually free, safe, and portable, the rubber-band apparatus can be a beautiful physical conditioner. First, you must get an inner tube from a passenger car or truck tire. Generally, service stations and tire shops just discard them, but many stations will be glad to give you one or sell one for a nominal price.

Once you have your inner tube, you will have to cut out the bands. This is relatively easy to do with a good pair of scissors. Cut each band about an inch or an inch-and-a-half wide. Because you're cutting a circle up into bands, you'll have to waste now and then to square off your cuts. I prefer to cut through the entire tube rather than to try and meet myself coming around. Cut straight across both surfaces.

Joining the bands into a working length is very easy. Generally, five or six bands make a good working length, although some prefer only three. Regardless of your preference, you may use the rubber band for a whole series of exercises, particularly for the arms and shoulders.

Biceps Exercise

(Strengthening)

When doing the biceps or "curl" exercise with the rubber bands, be sure the rubber band is securely back under the arch of your foot. Your forearm should be at a right angle to your upper arm, and the elbow must *not* rest on the hip. With your palm up and clenched on the band, raise your forearm and curl it up, bringing your clenched fist to your shoulder. Up and down, up and down. If it is too easy, shorten the rubber band. Repetitions should start at 5 and increase to 10 or 15.

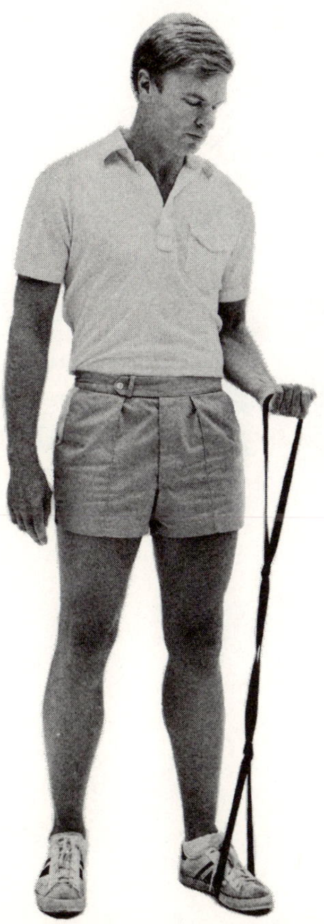

1 Place bottom loop of rubber band securely under arch of foot, grip top loop in upturned fist.

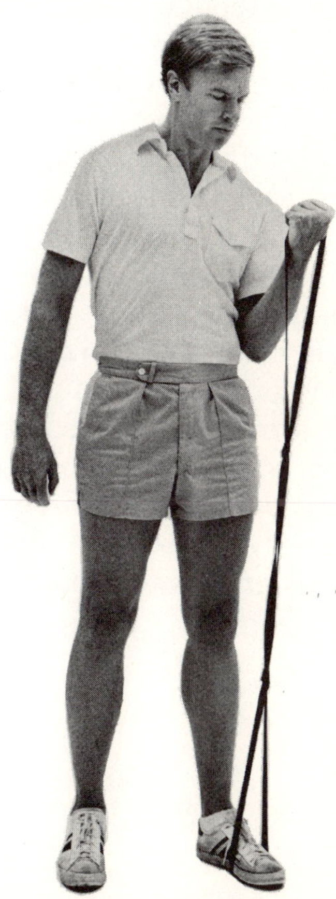

2 Curl arm up, down, up, down, at least 5 times for each arm. Later, increase to 10 or 15.

Chest Exercise

(Strengthening)

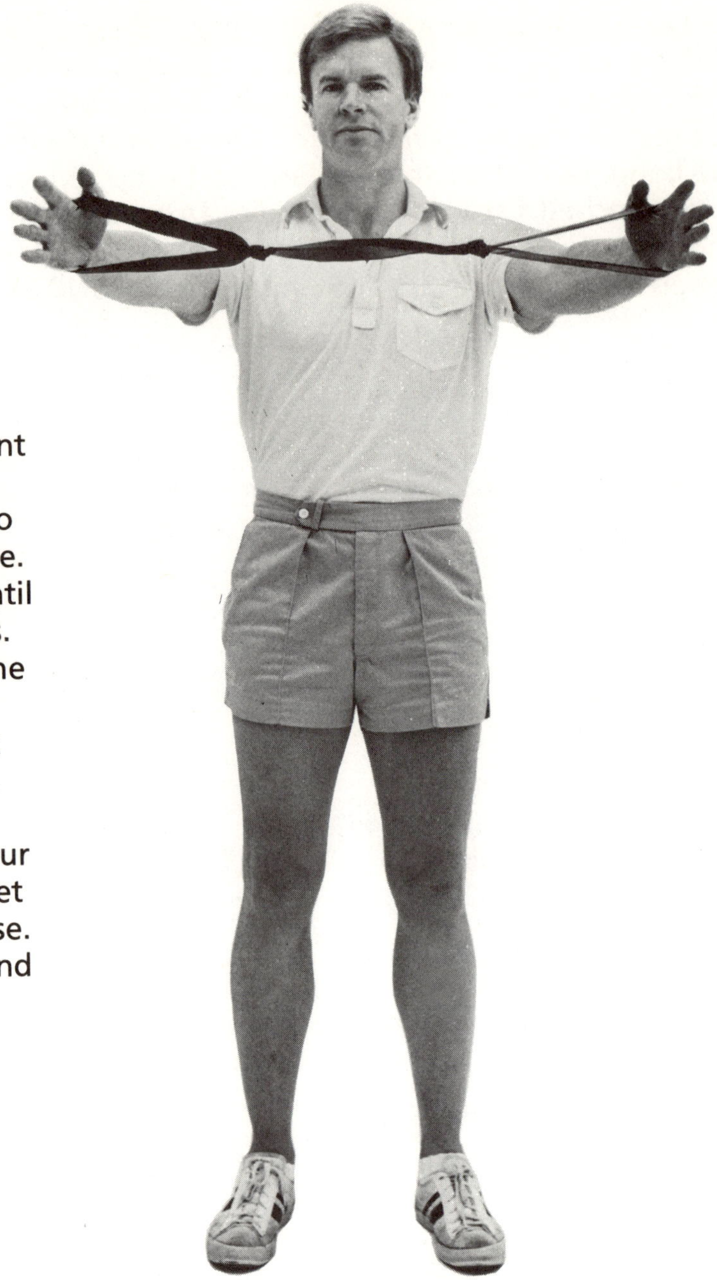

Start the chest exercise with both arms fully extended straight in front of you and your hands touching together. Affix the rubber band to your hands, as shown in the picture. Slowly spread your arms apart, until they are straight out at your sides. Think of a clock, lying face up on the floor in front of you. At the beginning, the hands of the clock (your two arms) are at 12 o'clock. When the exercise is completed, your left arm is at 9 o'clock, and your right arm is at 3 o'clock. Do not let your arms bend during this exercise. You may have to add a rubber band if the resistance is too much.

1 Grasp either end of rubber band with your arms extended straight in front of you.

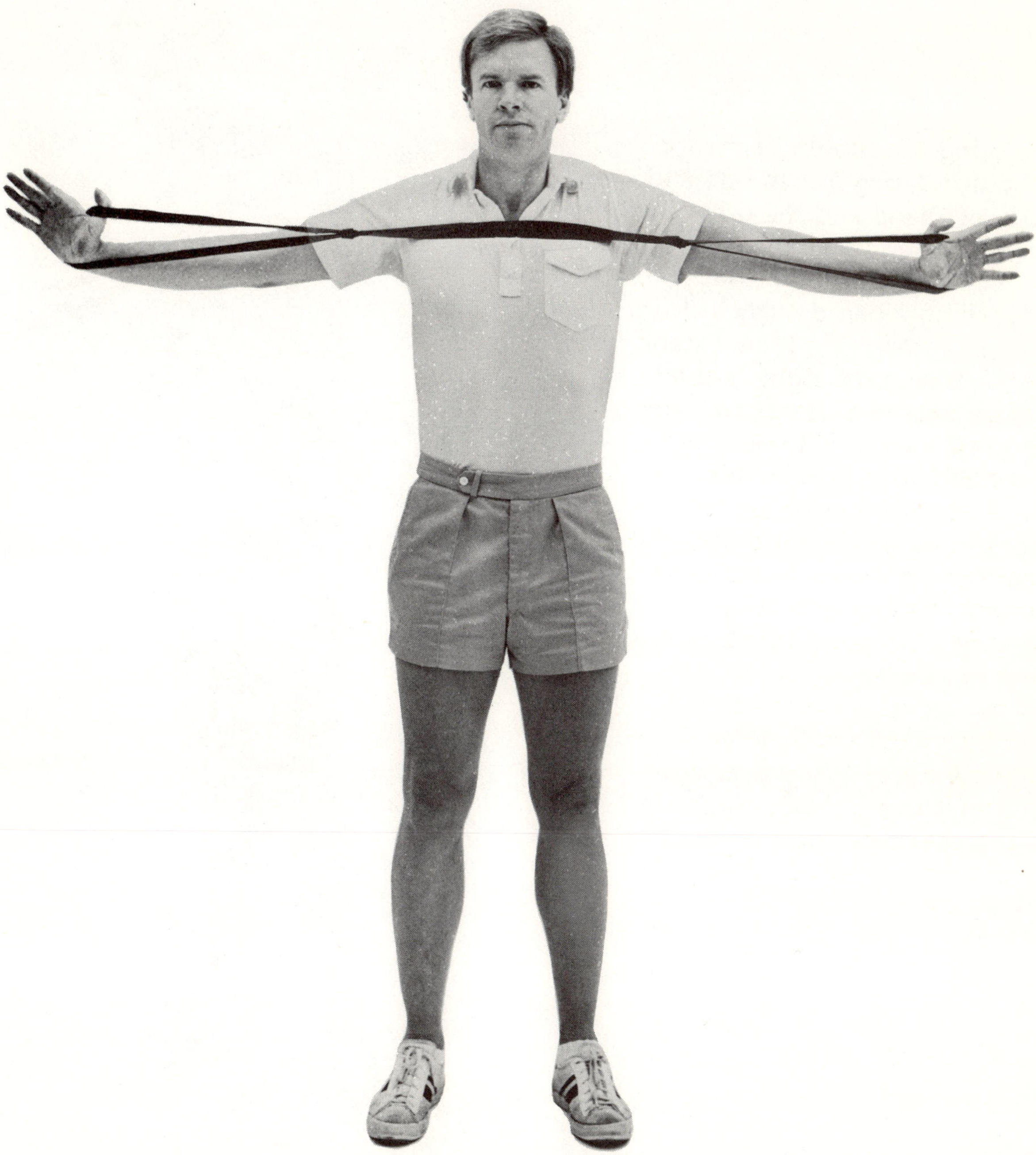

2 **Slowly bring arms back, keeping them straight, until arms are completely spread.**

Shoulders Exercise

(Strengthening)

When using the rubber bands for the shoulders, begin with one end in your left hand and the other in your right. Flip the bands over your back, and simply pretend that you are punching a bag directly in front of you, one hand at a time. Extend right, back with the right, extend left, back with the left, 15 or more times with each arm. Be sure to fully extend your arms in this exercise. Here are some additional exercises you can do with rubber bands. Remember to always keep your back straight and, when anchoring a band, be sure that it is anchored securely.

Additional rubber-band exercises (not illustrated) are described on pages 102–104.

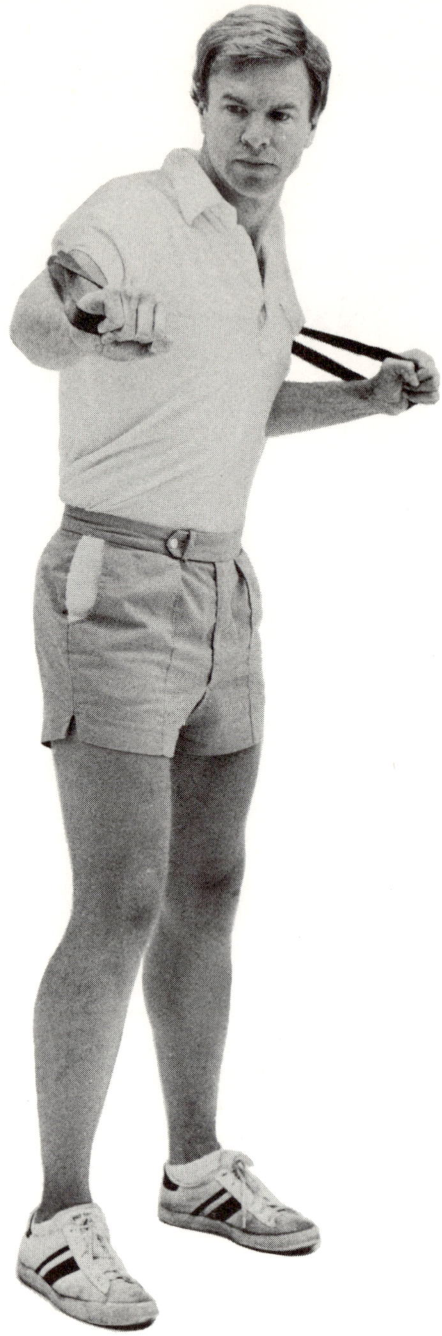

1 **Flip the rubber band over your head so that it rests on your shoulders.**

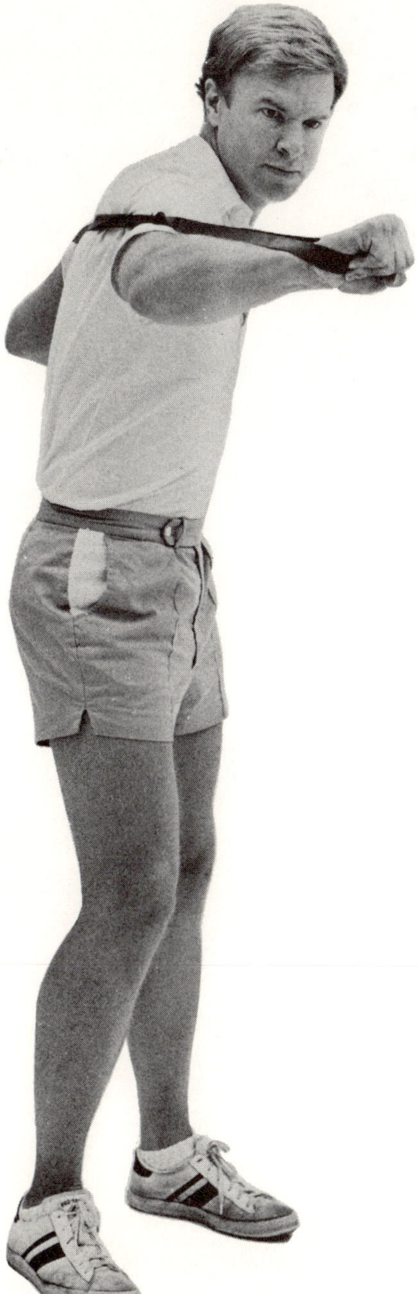

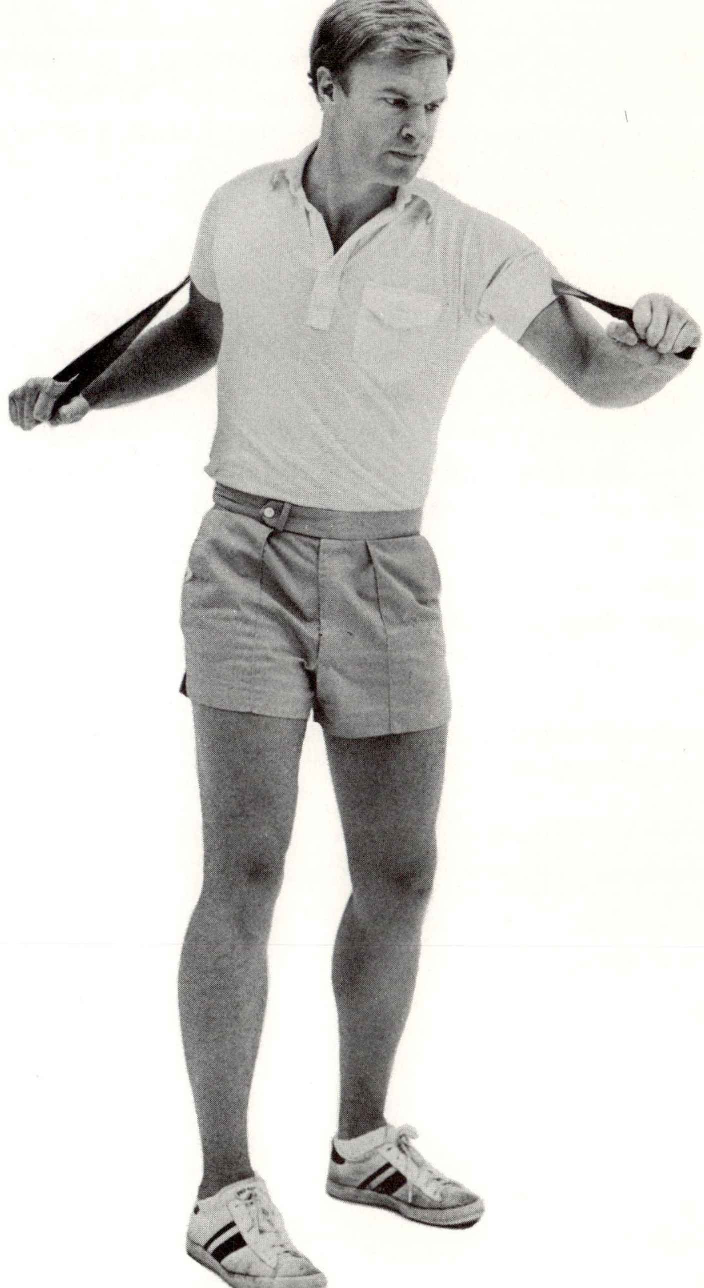

2 Pretend you are punching a bag directly in front of you, one fist at a time.

3 As you punch out with one arm, you draw back the other. Fully extend each arm.

Double Curl

(Strengthening)

If you really enjoy the rubber band program, here is an advanced exercise. You'll need a second rubber band made of three or four individual bands, just like your first one. You will also require a piece of old broomstick three feet long. Place your left foot in the bottom loop of one band and your right foot in the bottom loop of the other band. Place the broomstick in front of you with one end in the left top loop and the other end in the right top loop. Your forearms should be at right angles to your upper arms, and your elbows should *not* be on your hips. Curl both arms upward together.

This is a *double curl* exercise. If it is too easy, move the broomstick down to the next loop. Keep your back and legs straight throughout this exercise. Look straight ahead while curling upward. Start with 10 repetitions, and increase repetitions as it becomes easier to perform. You can also increase resistance with the size of the rubber bands as well as their length. The wider the band, the greater the resistance.

Overhead Press

(Strengthening)

Another advanced exercise is the Overhead Press. Start as if you were going to do the double curl described above. Now, with your palms facing *down* on the stick, raise the stick up to eye level and continue to press upward until both arms are fully extended straight above your head. You may need to add yet another band to perform this exercise. Be sure that the bands are well back on your feet and that the tension is not great enough to snap a band when you raise the stick. (They smart when they break!) Begin with 5 repetitions, and add as you are able. This is a good exercise for those who cannot do the doorway press because they are too short.

Pullover

(Strengthening)

On the floor, place two chains of rubber bands side by side. Anchor the last loop of each securely to the leg of a heavy chair, table, or dresser. Place the broomstick through the last loop of the free end of each rubber-band chain (just as you did for the curl or the press). Lie on your back on the floor, facing away from the dresser. With arms extended back, grasp the broomstick. Pull your arms up and forward, keeping your arms straight. Be sure the bands are well anchored. Pull as far forward as you can, keeping your arms straight. If resistance is too great, move closer to the point where the bands are anchored. Begin with 5 repetitions. Increase as you are able.

Ankle Rotation

(Strengthening)

Anchor one end of the rubber band on the leg of a dresser, heavy table, or bedstead. Place yourself in a chair facing this object. Hook the other end of the rubber band on the top of your foot, and extend your leg with your toes pointing straight up. Back the chair far enough away so as to put the rubber band under tension. Now, rotate your foot in a circular motion. Careful, don't let the band slip off; keep those toes up. Your ankle will tire rather quickly. Stop and transfer to the other ankle. Alternate back and forth 2 or 3 times. Ten seconds of rotating per ankle will probably be enough to start with. Alternate, giving equal attention to each ankle.

The Do's and Don'ts for Fitness

The selection of Do's and Don'ts that follows is not by any means to be regarded as a complete list. Far from it. Presented here are prescriptions, admonitions, and warnings that, when unheeded, have often resulted in misfortune or something much worse.

Following these Do's and Don'ts will greatly reduce the number of misfortunes that you should encounter through your own carelessness, ignorance, blundering, or having been born under the wrong sign (or on a Tuesday).

We're finishing up on a somewhat lighter note because, frankly, if you cannot relax about this program, you've already put an impossible burden on yourself. Relax and enjoy this unique approach to being fit. Being faithful to your routines and being stern and serious about it are not necessarily connected. Finally, be *patient* with yourself. It took you a long time to get soft, flabby, breathless, and weak. You're not going to overcome this overnight or in a fortnight or two. Just rejoice, knowing you're on the way to fitness!

The Do's

DO select a chair that will permit you to sit in it rather than seeking to evict you. What kind of chair is a good chair? One in which your back can and does remain straight. In a good recliner, for example, your back is straight even if the chair is tilted. Beware of all chairs in which you cannot reach the back with your back because the chair seat is so deep. This causes you to slump, with resulting stress and strain to the lower back.

DO keep your back straight when lifting, sweeping, mopping, and other related chores. Making the handles longer on these implements will make it much easier to stand erect while performing the task. The handle that reaches your chin is far better than the one that stops at your chest or armpit.

DO always stay close to your vacuum cleaner. Move your feet, rather than reaching with your arms and bending at the waist. Move around; your feet aren't nailed to the floor. When vacuuming stairs with an upright cleaner, lock it in the upright position and start on the top stair. Stand one step below the one you are vacuuming, and you'll be able to stand erect through the whole flight as you descend the stairs. Watch your step, though; you're descending back first. DO keep the stairs clear at all times!

DO adjust your ironing board so that you can sit while you iron. This is much more restful and won't affect your ironing at all. If you can't adjust your ironing board, you may be able to sit on something high, like a stool, as you iron.

DO stand on a stool when you need to reach up high for something. Never stand on the seat of a folding chair.

DO count calories; they do count.

DO wear shoes that are your actual size—not what you think your size should be. If you're a woman, remember that high heels not only affect your balance but can cause a backache.

DO use a night light. You'll stumble a lot less and reduce the chances of being unfit by reason of accident.

DO fall in love with water as your favorite snack. Water has no calories, caffeine, or sugar in it.

DO observe the program each and every day in every way that you can, especially beyond the time you allow for specific exercises. You can usually find stairs to the next floor, and take them two at a time instead of waiting for the elevator. In short, whenever you can exercise, do so.

DO take a relaxation break; do the tension release exercises several times a day, whether you feel tense or not.

DO cut down on your intake of caffeine. All of the cola drinks (except for new "decaffeinated" cola) are heavy with caffeine, whether they are diet colas or not. Some noncola soft drinks now contain added caffeine (look at the label). Caffeine is a stimulant, and a little goes a long way. Use decaffeinated coffee whenever possible.

DO avoid excessive salt in your food. It can lead to high blood pressure. Forget to put the salt shaker on the table. Most of us consume far more salt than the body needs.

DO moderate your drinking, if you drink at all. Apart from the bad effects of too much alcohol, there is the matter of calories. There are an enormous amount of calories in a small volume of liquor, although the new low-calorie wines and beers do make a difference.

DO elevate your baby's crib so that the mattress is waist high (your waist). When you drop the crib side to take baby out, your arms will be able to grasp your baby without your having to bend at all. Do not just raise the mattress; if you do, your youngster might find it too easy to climb out. Find a stable way to lengthen the legs—and save your back.

The Don'ts

DON'T participate in any sport without loosening up first! Do so with the stretching exercises described in this book.

DON'T ski without observing preconditioning, particularly for the knees and for general suppleness.

DON'T sit on a toboggan unless you are on a prepared toboggan run. Compression fractures of vertebrae occur all too frequently while tobogganing. If you must, kneel on a good pad rather than sitting when you are tobogganing on one of nature's unprepared slopes. And keep your hands inside.

DON'T ever use a power mower without good shoes on or with your legs uncovered. That whirling blade can slice a toe or turn gravel into bullets. Power mowers injure thousands of persons each year.

DON'T lift with your legs apart and straight while bending at the waist. Drop down to the object by bending your knees and keeping your back straight. Look straight ahead, and this will help to keep your back straight.

DON'T attempt to push a car alone; get a crew and push together. Better yet, use another vehicle or a tow truck.

DON'T use the cellar, attic, or other stairs as extra shelves.

DON'T weed your garden by straddling the rows, bending at the waist, and keeping the legs straight. Always bend with the knees.

DON'T ever climb a ladder of any kind with anything in your hands. Grab the ladder with both hands.

DON'T ever step on the top edge of a bathtub. If you're not sure of yourself, keep a sturdy chair near the tub, and grasp the chair when you enter or leave. Some people are very unsteady on one leg, even for the moment it takes to step into or out of a tub.

DON'T be a weekend athlete if you're not willing to observe a conditioning program every day, as described in this book.

DON'T depend on jogging for year-round exercise. Weather, darkness, and other conditions often make it inadvisable to jog. You can always skip rope, run in place, or fast dance, and, if you do so with real vigor, you'll do as much (or more) for your heart muscle than you will by moderate jogging.

Epilogue

One of the most prevalent and hurtful echoes from the PE programs of yesteryear is the idea that unless you're really suffering you're not going to achieve fitness. Nonsense. You are *not* a professional athlete fighting for your livelihood within the arena of cutthroat physical competition. Forget all that. There's more than enough suffering in this world without making an effort to add to the stockpile of misery and pain. On the other hand, a little more awareness of where your muscles are won't bring any permanent pain or lasting remorse.

Enjoy your program, and try to apply it every day in every way that is relevant. Remember, functional fitness is concern for your well-being, both when you're exercising and whenever you are putting your body under stress in a variety of simple and mundane tasks. Functional fitness determines the way you sit, walk, lift, sweep, shovel, rake, weed, iron, and perform countless other tasks.

Begin Each Day with These Exercises

—Your 15 Minutes for Fitness

Here, as a memory aid, are shown in order 10 exercises for you to do every weekday morning, followed by a list of optional morning exercises. All are pictured and described in detail on pages 40–71. The numbers in parentheses indicate the specific page or pages on which the exercise appears.

If you take a minute or so for each of the ten illustrated exercises, you'll be off to a healthy start.

1 Knee to Chest/Ear (40–41)

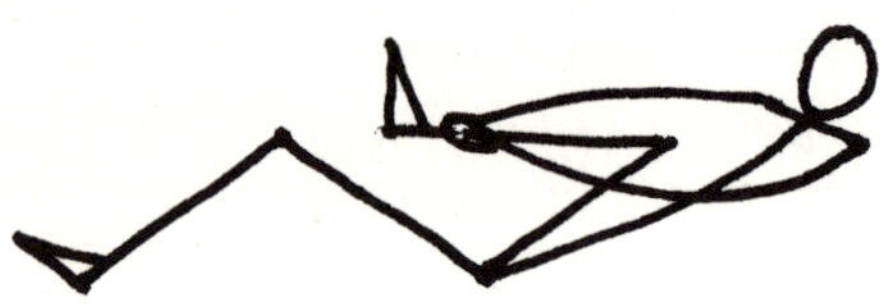

2 Sitback (42–47)

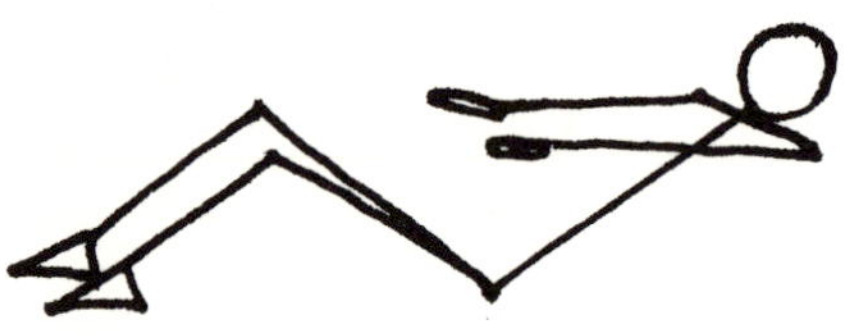

3 Supine Stretch (48)

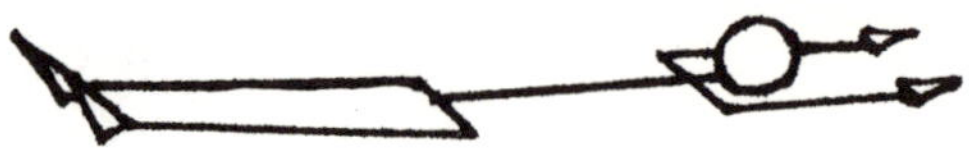

4 Praying Press (49)

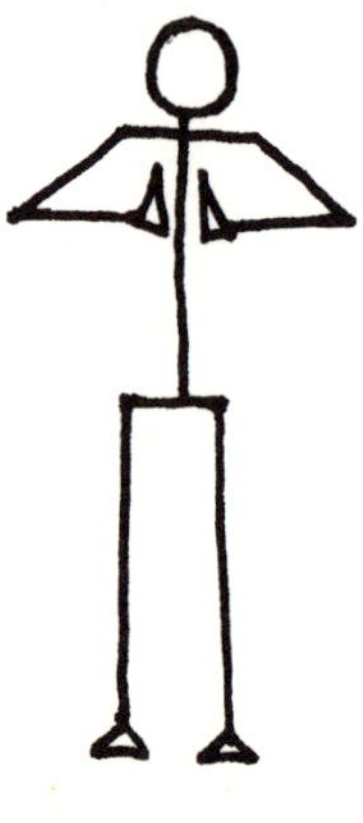

5 **Neck Pull (50–51)**

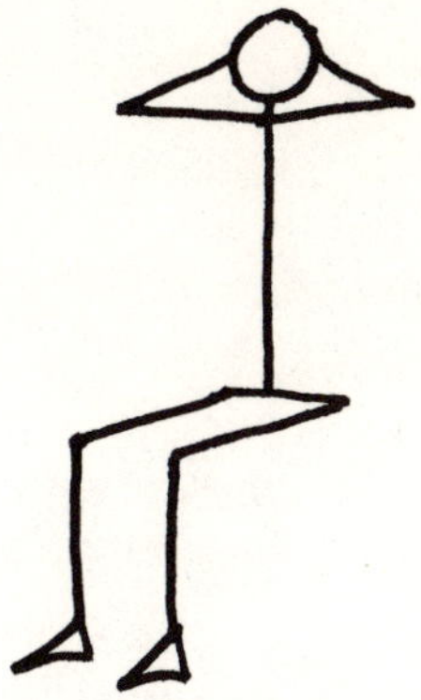

8 **Doorway Press (62)**

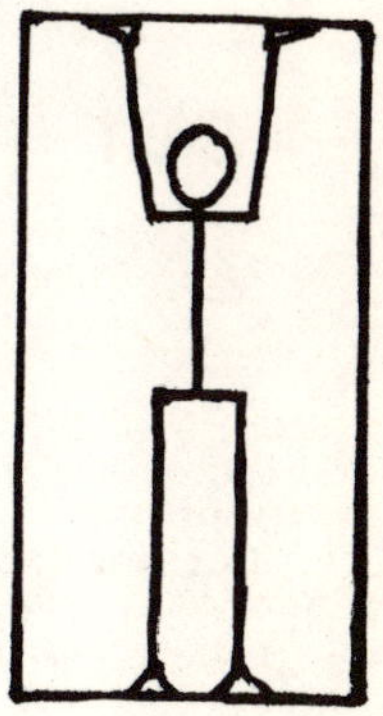

6 **Dancer's Exercise (58–59)**

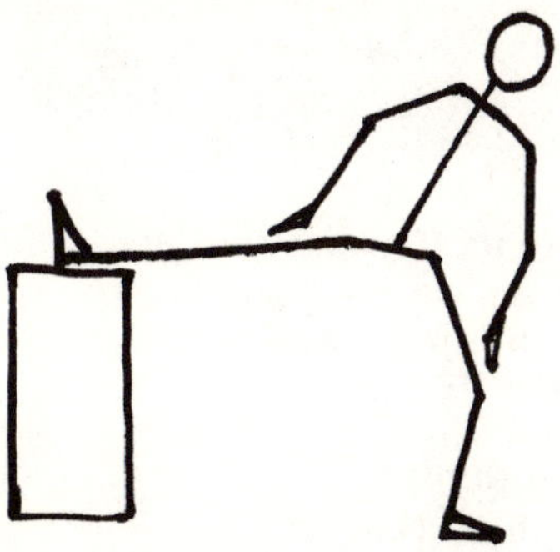

9 **Push-Ups (64–69)**

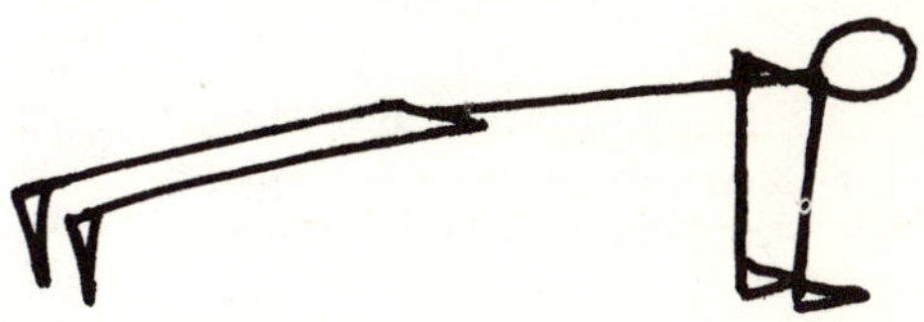

7 **Toe-Ups (60–61)**

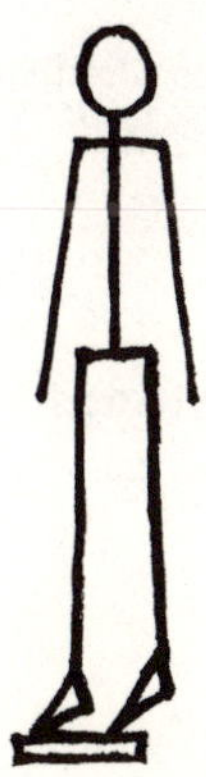

10 **Leg Press-Ups (70–71)**

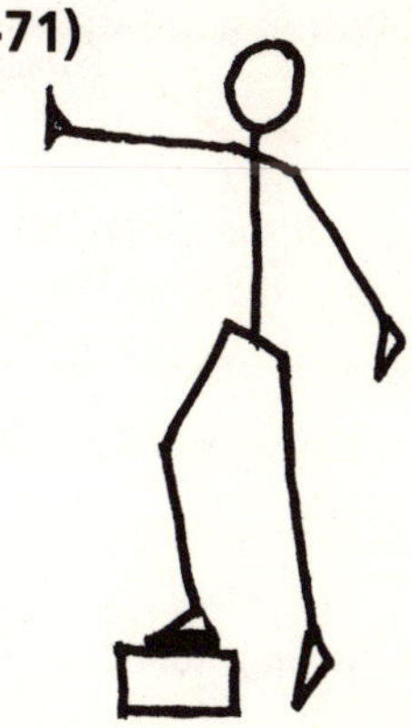

Optionals

Gathering Marbles (52–53)
Crumpling Newspaper (54–55)
Bear Hug (56–57)
Arm Circles (61)
Wall Sit (63)

Exercises for Each Part of the Body

Shoulders
Doorway Press (62), Push-Ups (64–69), Shoulders Exercise (100–101)

Arms
Arm Circles (61), Doorway Press (62), Push-Ups (64–69), Biceps Exercise (97)

Bust/Chest
Praying Press (49), Bear Hug (56–57), Arm Circles (61), Push-Ups (64–69)

Waist
Eat Less!

Buttocks/Hips
Wall Sit (63), Fast Dancing, Rope Skipping, Running in Place, Walking

Thighs
Wall Sit (63), Bicycling, Fast Dancing, Rope Skipping, Running in Place

Knees
Leg Press-Ups (70–71), NO DEEP KNEE BENDS

Calves
Toe-Ups (60–61), Wall Sit (63), Fast Dancing, Rope Skipping, Running in Place, Walking

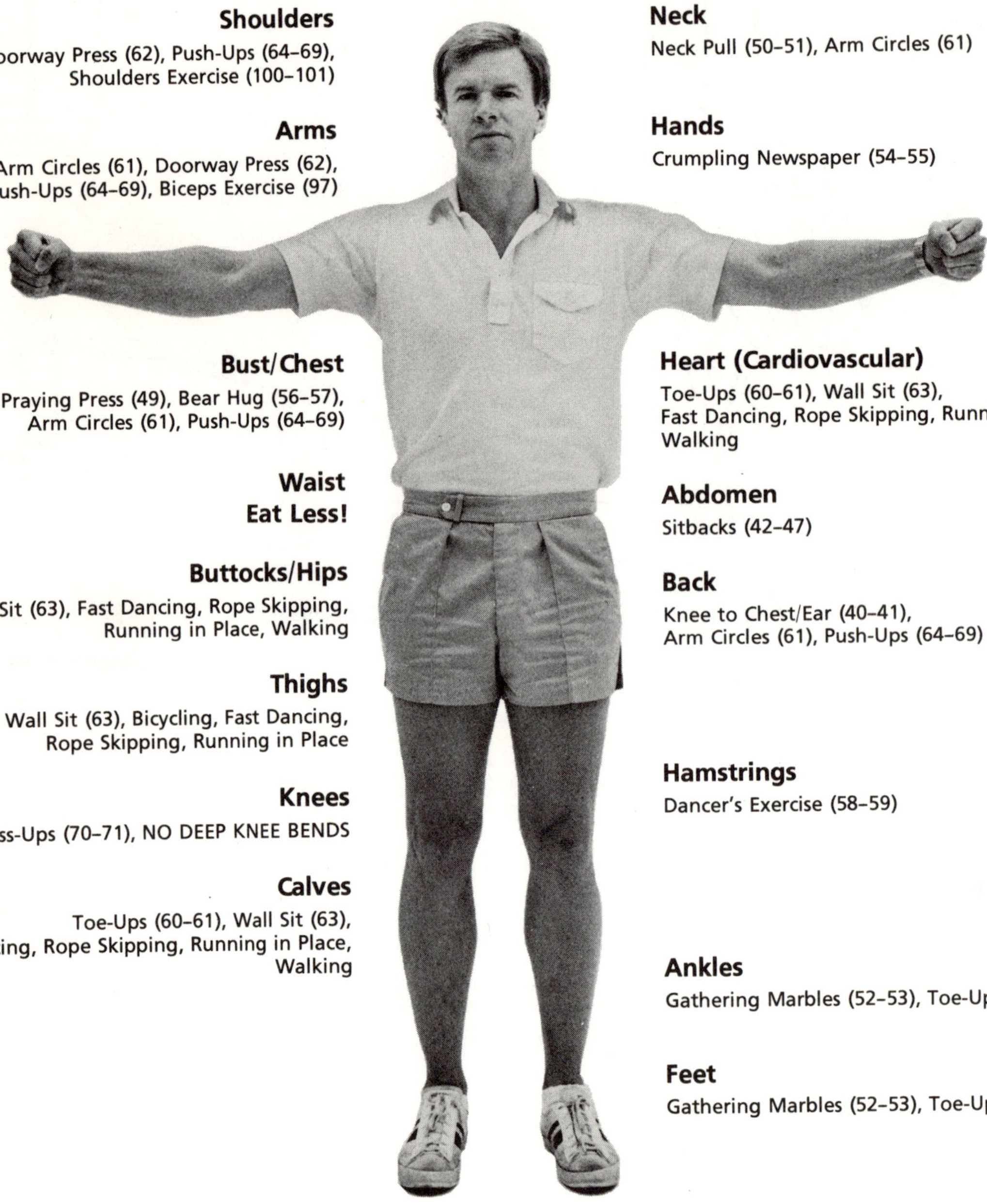

Neck
Neck Pull (50–51), Arm Circles (61)

Hands
Crumpling Newspaper (54–55)

Heart (Cardiovascular)
Toe-Ups (60–61), Wall Sit (63), Fast Dancing, Rope Skipping, Running in Place, Walking

Abdomen
Sitbacks (42–47)

Back
Knee to Chest/Ear (40–41), Arm Circles (61), Push-Ups (64–69)

Hamstrings
Dancer's Exercise (58–59)

Ankles
Gathering Marbles (52–53), Toe-Ups (60–61)

Feet
Gathering Marbles (52–53), Toe-Ups (60–61)